What You Can Do
to Prevent
Diabetes

What You Can Do to Prevent Diabetes

Simple Changes to Improve Your Life

Annette Maggi, M.S., R.D.

Jackie Boucher, M.S., R.D., C.D.E.

JOHN WILEY & SONS, INC.

New York • Chichester • Weinheim • Brisbane • Singapore • Toronto

Published by John Wiley & Sons, Inc.
Published simultaneously in Canada
Design and composition by Navta Associates, Inc.

The information contained in this book is not intended to serve as a replacement for professional medical advice. Any use of the information in this book is at the reader's discretion. The author and the publisher specifically disclaim any and all liability arising directly or indirectly from the use or application of any information contained in this book. A health care professional should be consulted regarding your specific situation.

Library of Congress Cataloging-in-Publication Data:
Maggi, Annette.
  What you can do to prevent diabetes : simple changes to improve your life / Annette Maggi, Jackie Boucher.
    p.   cm.
  Includes index.
  ISBN 0-471-34796-5 (paper)
  1. Non-insulin-dependent diabetes—Prevention.   2. Non-insulin-dependent diabetes—Popular works.   I. Boucher, Jackie.   II. Title.

RC662.18.M345   2000
616.4'6205—dc21   99-052765

This book is dedicated to all those who are willing to believe that it's never too late to change and that simple changes can bring big results.

✌ Contents ∾

∿ Introduction ∿

For years, the fact that you can prevent heart disease and cancer has been much discussed. All it takes, it seems, is eating less fat and more fruits and vegetables, being more active physically, and living a smoke-free life.

But diabetes? No one ever said you could prevent diabetes.

Actually, you can. More and more research is accumulating every day to prove it. For example, more than 27 percent of new cases of type 2 diabetes could be prevented if we didn't gain weight over the years. Exercising can also help—incidence of type 2 diabetes is 30 to 50 percent lower in those who exercise regularly. And that is only the beginning. There are many actions we can take to decrease the odds of getting diabetes.

If you've picked up this book, you're obviously thinking that diabetes may affect you in the future. Perhaps you've had a parent or a sibling die from complications related to diabetes. Or maybe this disease has come up in a conversation with your doctor because you had a blood glucose test that was a little high. No matter why you're interested in preventing diabetes, you've picked up the right resource.

Because this is such a new area of health and wellness, the number of resources available to tell us how to prevent diabetes has been limited. For this reason, *What You Can Do to Prevent Diabetes: Simple Changes to Improve Your Life* came to be. It is the guide for all of us interested in living without this disease. It is filled with small changes you can easily incorporate into your daily life to lower your chances of getting diabetes. *What You Can Do to Prevent Diabetes* is written in a format that is useful for busy people—short sections of information that can be read in a few spare minutes, maybe over breakfast, or while pedaling on the exercise bike, or while waiting at a doctor's office.

There are three key steps to preventing diabetes: 1. managing your weight, 2. getting active, and 3. building healthier eating habits. All three are covered here. Yet, making changes in these areas of your life is often affected by other factors. As a result, this book gives you insight into finding life balance and an understanding of the change process and how to really be successful at it. It also shows you how to involve the entire family in diabetes prevention and, in the final part, gives ideas on how to maintain positive new lifestyle habits.

If you think that diabetes can't happen to you, think again. Sixteen million Americans have diabetes and half of us don't even know it. Odds are that another 20 million of us will get diabetes, yet we don't think it will ever happen to us. But it can, and unfortunately, there's currently no cure for diabetes. Prevention is the only choice.

❧ PART ONE ☙

Rate Your Risk for Developing Diabetes

Most likely, we all have at least one family member, friend, or co-worker who has diabetes. Do we really understand what it means to have diabetes? Are there people who are more prone to getting this disease? Could you be one of them? Although we can't change our parents, our race, our age, or our sex, the good news is we can make lifestyle changes that can prevent us from getting diabetes.

~: | :~

Will You Get Diabetes?

Have you ever really thought about diabetes? Have you seriously thought that you could develop this disease? Most people think about cancer and heart disease—and how to prevent them—but what about diabetes?

If you've never thought about it before now, you're not alone. In fact, three-quarters of those over the age of 45 don't know whether they have diabetes. Yet more than 16 million of us have the disease. So how can you tell if you're likely to be one of the people who get it? The key is to look at factors that increase your chances of getting diabetes—the *risk factors*. Read the following statements and circle those that apply to you:

Risk Factors for Diabetes

- I'm over the age of 45.

- One of my parents, brothers, or sisters has diabetes.

- I'm a woman who gave birth to a baby weighing more than nine pounds at birth, or I have a history of gestational diabetes.

- My doctor has told me that I have impaired fasting glucose or impaired glucose tolerance.

- My heritage is African American, Hispanic/Latino, Native American, Asian American, or Pacific Islander.

- I have high blood pressure.

- I have a low high-density lipoprotein (HDL, the "good" cholesterol) level or a high triglyceride level.

- My weight is 20 percent or more above the recommended weight for my height.

- I don't exercise much or I'm not very active on a day-to-day basis.

Now look back over the list. The more statements you've circled, the greater your chances of developing diabetes during your life.

When you look over the list, you may notice that some of the risk factors are beyond your control, such as age, having a family history of diabetes, giving birth to a large baby, or your heritage. This could make you feel like there's no chance of preventing diabetes. But look at the list again and notice all of the factors you can work to control, like your weight and activity level.

Although having several uncontrollable risk factors significantly increases your chances of developing diabetes, changing those factors that are within your control, like weight and exercise, can increase the likelihood that you'll live into your golden years without ever getting this chronic disease.

~: 2 :~

Understanding Diabetes

Without having a *reason* to do something, most of us won't take any action. At this point, you may know you're at risk for developing diabetes, but what does that really mean? What is this disease called *diabetes* anyway?

Simply put, diabetes is a chronic disease in which the body can't properly use the food we eat; the body doesn't make enough insulin or can't use it properly to change food into energy. Normally, the digestive system changes most food into glucose—the body's preferred energy source. Once the food is digested, glucose enters the bloodstream, causing blood glucose levels to rise. Glucose is carried in the blood cells to be used as fuel, but insulin needs to be available for the glucose to be absorbed into the cells. *Insulin* is a hormone made and secreted by the *pancreas*, a gland near the stomach. In response to the rising blood glucose level, the pancreas releases insulin into the bloodstream, causing the glucose to enter the cells so blood glucose levels return to normal.

If we have diabetes, however, our body doesn't work like it should. There are problems with how much insulin our pancreas makes and how well our cells use the available insulin. They've become insulin resistant. As a result, the glucose can't get into our cells to provide energy and our blood glucose levels remain high. Eventually, because our body isn't getting the fuel it needs, we start to feel tired and hungry. These problems in our body's handling of glucose occur gradually over time. In fact, most people diagnosed with diabetes have had it for a while—often up to seven years—without even knowing it!

This kind of diabetes, in which the body makes some insulin but can't use it properly, is called type 2 diabetes. About

90 to 95 percent of people with diabetes have this type. It most often occurs in overweight adults and some overweight teens. Managing type 2 diabetes involves losing weight, leading an active lifestyle, and sometimes taking oral medications or insulin injections.

The other type of diabetes—type 1—usually occurs in people under age 20, affecting only 5 to 10 percent of all people who are diagnosed with diabetes. People with type 2 diabetes still make insulin, but those with type 1 diabetes produce little or no insulin and require daily injections to survive. Scientists are still working to determine if type 1 diabetes is preventable.

Both types of diabetes are serious, requiring long-term lifestyle changes to treat the disease and to prevent complications of the disease that can occur, such as eye, kidney, nerve, and heart damage. So, knowing that you could prevent a disease that could cause you health problems in the not-so-distant future, aren't you ready to take action?

~: 3 :~

Diabetes Develops over Time

Many illnesses—a virus, food poisoning, or chicken pox—strike suddenly. We wake up one morning and find that we are sick. But this isn't true of diabetes. It doesn't just happen overnight or over a few days. We can actually have diabetes for years before really feeling sick or before our health care provider diagnoses it.

But how can this be? How can we walk around for years feeling okay, not knowing we're sick? Here's how.

Although no one knows the exact cause, it is known that age, genetics, and lifestyle habits can affect whether or not you develop type 2 diabetes. Over a period of years, these factors can slowly contribute to your body's inability to produce or to use insulin. When this happens, a doctor may diagnose you with either impaired fasting glucose or impaired glucose tolerance—meaning you're having problems using insulin the right way. These are the first steps leading up to a diabetes diagnosis. A simple test called a fasting glucose test, which is administered at a health care provider's office, can tell you if you have either one of these initial stages of diabetes.

So when does full-blown diabetes happen? How will you know when you have it? Some of the symptoms you may experience are weakness, fatigue, excessive hunger, extreme thirst, frequent urination, changes in vision, or persistent infections. At this point, because your body's ability to produce insulin or to use it appropriately becomes even more impaired, you start to feel sick. Often, however, you may not even know you have diabetes until you go to see your doctor for a routine physical. Many individuals don't experience any of the common symptoms.

So what can you do? If you know you are at risk for getting diabetes, or if you are already in the initial stages, visit your health care provider regularly. If you're 45 years of age or older and have risk factors for diabetes, have a fasting glucose test every three years to make sure you haven't developed diabetes. At the same time, focus on what you can do to prevent diabetes or to reverse the initial stages, such as impaired fasting glucose or impaired glucose tolerance. The key is starting now, not later. By managing your weight, leading an active lifestyle, and following healthy eating patterns, you can turn back time and prevent diabetes.

~: 4 :~

Stack the Odds in Your Favor

With the fast pace of life today, it's common for us to take chances. For instance, the weather might be bad, but we venture out into a storm because we have so much to do at work that we can't afford to miss a day. We don't think about staying home even though it may be safer. We don't consider the odds that something could happen to us or to our cars.

Our decision about whether to work to prevent diabetes may follow a similar unfortunate path. We may decide to take our chances and to deal with the consequences of diabetes, instead of trying to change our lifestyle right now to prevent it. "It won't happen to me," right? Yet every minute, one person is diagnosed with diabetes, and you could be next—depending on the number of risk factors you have. If you're a betting person, you'd be smart to stack the odds against developing diabetes in your favor now because there's no cure for this disease once you get it. The best chance to live your life without diabetes is to work to prevent it.

Once you get diabetes, the odds for additional complications also work against you. If blood glucose levels are uncontrolled over the years, you can develop eye disease, heart and blood vessel disease that can lead to a heart attack or a stroke, kidney disease, and nerve disease. Skin, feet, and dental problems are also common complications of diabetes.

Although you might be betting on the fact that diabetes won't happen to you, you are probably unaware of your chances for getting long-term complications from diabetes. But the following statistics may change your mind:

- Diabetes is the leading cause of new blindness in people

20 to74 years of age. Each year 12,000 to 24,000 people with diabetes lose their sight.

- About 10 to 20 percent of people with diabetes develop kidney problems.

- People with diabetes are two to four times more likely to have heart disease . . . and their rates of death from heart disease are two to four times higher than in adults without diabetes. People with diabetes are also two to four times more likely to have a stroke.

- Approximately 60 to 70 percent of people with diabetes have mild to severe forms of nerve damage, which, in severe forms, can lead to lower-limb amputation. Each year more than 56,000 people with diabetes lose a foot or a leg.

So given the numbers, do you still want to roll the dice without putting the odds in your favor? It's not only diabetes you'll be preventing but also all the health complications this disease can bring. Once you've got the facts, the choice between getting this chronic and sometimes debilitating disease and not getting it is very clear. Remember these frightening statistics, and change the odds in your favor.

~: 5 :~

Preventing Diabetes
Doesn't Have to Be a Mystery

Everyone loves mysteries. Who did it? Why? Where? How? There have been hundreds, probably thousands, of mystery books written. There have been successful television shows, such as *Murder She Wrote* or *Unsolved Mysteries*. There are even murder mystery games.

So what is it about mysteries that we love? Most likely, it's finding the trail of clues that lead to solving the puzzle. Discovering the facts that lead you to preventing diabetes is no different. Once you see the facts and understand how they fit together, the mystery is solved. The only difference is that at the end of your detective work, you're the one who needs to act to prevent diabetes from happening.

Just what are the facts? Well for starters, people who lead an active lifestyle can decrease their chances of getting diabetes by 30 to 50 percent. At least 27 percent of the people diagnosed with diabetes might have been able to prevent it if they had avoided gaining weight. So managing your weight and increasing your level of physical activity are two crucial steps in your diabetes prevention efforts. What you eat also matters. If you eat more calories than you expend in exercise and day-to-day activities, you gain weight.

So, mystery solved. The facts show that our activity level, the way we manage our weight, and what we eat can and will make a difference in our plan to prevent diabetes. The detective work may be done, but the action is just beginning. It's up to you to change your lifestyle for the better.

Simple Changes Journal

What can you do *today* to better understand your chances of getting diabetes?

What can you do *this week* to better understand your chances of getting diabetes?

What can you do *this month* to better understand your chances of getting diabetes?

◡ PART TWO ◡

Make Lifestyle Changes That Last

To prevent diabetes, you need to exercise, manage your weight, and eat nutritious foods. Sounds simple, doesn't it? If only it really were that simple. We can't develop new lifestyle habits overnight, yet we expect changes to happen quickly, almost magically. If we want to do something, we just do it, right? Wrong! Behavior change isn't an event—something that happens or doesn't happen—it's a process. We can't build the habits necessary to prevent diabetes until we understand the change process and are ready to change our current lifestyle habits to healthier ones. Before you just jump in and tell yourself you're going to start exercising and eating better, you need to learn how to make changes for lasting success. Change—it really is a good thing when it comes to preventing diabetes and building a healthier lifestyle.

❧ 6 ❧

How Ready Are You to Change?

Do you ever notice how most of us think and talk about changing a bad habit—such as smoking or watching television instead of getting active in the evening—but never actually make the change? We beat ourselves up about things like this all the time. We talk about having no willpower or motivation and call ourselves lazy. But do you know what? We should stop being so hard on ourselves. Why? Because we all change different behaviors at various rates.

According to James Prochaska, coauthor of the book *Changing for Good*, change doesn't happen in a straight line, always moving forward. Instead, sometimes we try to initiate a change, we move forward, but then we often slip backward—two steps forward, one step back. This is why we may be thinking about changing a habit but haven't actually done it yet. We're not at that point in the change process yet.

In the first stage of change—*precontemplation*—we're not even thinking about changing. For example, we may not be aware that our chances of developing diabetes are high. Often, at this stage, we say to ourselves, "I don't have a problem." We see no reason to change, so we continue to avoid the issue. We often rationalize our behavior or blame others. We might make statements such as, "You're the problem, not me," or "I can't change."

To move forward to the next stage, we need to become aware of the facts on why it's important to change, to learn the benefits of change, and to acknowledge that new behaviors make our lives feel different. For example, if we don't know how exercise prevents diabetes or if we don't know all the benefits we get from exercise, we may be less likely to consider fitting exercise into our schedule. Also, at first, we may feel awkward doing a new exercise or exercising at all, which may make us less apt to keep doing it. Any new habit can feel uncomfortable at first; but with time, it does become second nature.

Contemplation is the next step in the change process. Contemplators are seriously thinking about making a change in the next six months. At this point, we're still rationalizing the costs of a new habit, but at least we're starting to think that there could be benefits to doing things differently. Yet the rule of thumb is still "when in doubt, don't change."

If we listen to ourselves, we might hear: "I'll start when the time is right" or "Let me think about it" or "I'd like to, but . . ." We're still waiting for that magic moment to occur before beginning. In order to keep the momentum moving forward, we need to reinforce the positive benefits we'll experience and imagine how good we'll feel once we've made the changes.

Once we've contemplated change, decided that the positive outcomes outweigh the negatives, and decided to move forward, we're in the *preparation* stage—the midpoint of the process. We're intending to develop new habits in the next thirty days. We may have made some changes in the past but have not been successful at maintaining them. Often, we know what we want to do but aren't sure how to start.

At this stage, change at least feels doable. We might be saying to ourselves, "I'm ready to start" or "I will do this . . ." or "How do I go about changing ———?" When we've reached this stage, our plan helps us keep going forward; the lack of a plan sends us spiraling backward to contemplation. Here, it's important to continue to seek out information, to get support from others, to reinforce the positive benefits of change, and to set realistic goals.

When we're actively exercising, eating nutritious foods, or taking steps to manage stress, we're in the *action* stage. We have found the motivation, the commitment, the time, and the energy to put our health first. Change really starts to feel comfortable. At this point, we might be saying to ourselves, "I'm doing it" or "I know I can do it." To keep up the action, we need to continue to develop new skills, to build our self-confidence in doing the new behavior, and to reward ourselves for the changes we're making.

After six months of actively practicing a new behavior, we reach the next stage of change—*maintenance*. Once we achieve the desired behavior, we initially find that maintaining the new behavior takes a conscious effort. With repetition over time, we don't notice the effort—the behavior feels very natural. When we no longer need to think about the behavior at all, we have truly acquired a habit.

But change is a process. It takes time before a new behavior becomes a habit. Even in maintenance, we can expect minor setbacks—they are inevitable. The key is to pick up where we left off and to continue our new, healthier habits.

Now that you understand the process of behavior change, you might want to think about where you're at with the key lifestyle habits that can help you prevent diabetes, such as managing your weight or increasing your level of physical activity. If you're interested, make a list of the behavior changes you want to make (for example, start exercising, eat less fat, manage stress) on a sheet of paper, and next to the behavior change, write the stage of change in which you think you are for that behavior.

As you begin to outline the action steps you'll take to prevent diabetes, refer back to this list. When developing a health plan, it's best to focus on those behaviors you're still contemplating changing or preparing to change. Your goal is to eventually move into action for those behaviors. Once you do, you'll be one step closer to preventing diabetes.

~ 7 ~

Learn from Past Successes

It's easy to think about all the failures we've had. But we should also think about the successes—the things we've really done well, the positive improvements we've made, the new skills we've developed.

Reflecting on our experiences is helpful as we prepare to improve our lifestyle. It helps us to realize that we have been successful before and to understand how we dealt with failures. It results in increased self-confidence in our ability to make changes that can last.

We've all been successful at certain positive lifestyle behaviors at some time. Perhaps we used to go to the health club regularly to exercise, ate fruit for breakfast, or maintained a weight loss. What healthy lifestyle habits are you currently maintaining? Why are you able to continue them? What behavior changes have you made in the past that you were able to do only for a while before slipping back to old behaviors? What was different about your life then?

Now, if you want to learn more about your successes, you may want to take a sheet of paper and create two columns. In the first column, list the actions you're currently taking to improve your health and those you've done before. In the second column, next to each action, write all the reasons you've been successful at making a behavior change, even if it was only for a short time. For example, you scheduled exercise appointments, you cut up fruits and vegetables for snacking during the week, or you attended a support group. Once you have the action list completed, look it over very carefully. Some of the strategies you used in the past may be helpful as you try to make changes now and in the future.

∿ 8 ∿

Overcome Obstacles
on the Road to Change

Have you ever watched the movie or read the book *The Wizard of Oz*? When Dorothy's house lands in Oz after the tornado, all she wants to do is go home to Kansas. So the Munchkins tell her to follow the yellow brick road and find the Wizard who can help her.

In the end, she does get home, but have you ever thought about the barriers she experienced on her trip to Oz? The Wicked Witch of the West was a constant barrier because she wanted Dorothy's red slippers. The Scarecrow she met at the crossroads wasn't sure he could help her because he didn't believe he had a brain. The Cowardly Lion felt he wasn't brave, so didn't feel he could protect the group when the going got tough. The Tin Man, well, he didn't feel he had a heart. Each had set up barriers in their lives. In reality, they always had the abilities or skills, they just didn't see them.

We often see barriers when we try to change, and those barriers are generally what keep us from being successful. For most of us, common barriers to change are lack of time, resources, skills, or social support. You can take steps to overcome your barriers to success—you just need to plan and to believe you can do it.

If time is a barrier, you can shift priorities in your schedule or replace some time-wasting habits with positive lifestyle behaviors. Every day has twenty-four hours. Assuming that you work for eight hours and sleep for eight hours, what happens in the remaining eight hours of your day? Is it possible to exercise while you watch TV, to get up thirty minutes earlier in the morning to exercise, or to plan an exercise activity as a family outing? There are many ways to use your time to your advantage.

Lack of resources is another common barrier people create

for themselves. It doesn't take a health club membership to exercise, or body massages to relax, or expensive foods to eat healthfully. Access to these nice services make life easier, but they aren't necessary. You can walk with co-workers at lunchtime; learn some relaxation techniques to reduce stress, such as deep breathing, from books in the library; and shop at a farmer's market in the summer for fresh fruits and vegetables or buy frozen vegetables in the winter.

If you feel you don't have the skills you need to effect change, success can be difficult. If you think you aren't coordinated enough to exercise or underestimate your cooking abilities, you probably won't be good at either skill—just like the characters in *The Wizard of Oz*. The key is whether you think you can learn and then attempt to do so. One idea is to ask friends whom you admire for their exercise aptitude to teach you to play tennis, swim, or in-line skate. Take a cooking class or practice testing recipes until you feel comfortable preparing some new healthful meals. If you think you can do it, you will. To gain skills, write a list of the skills you have and the skills you want to develop; then think of people, classes, or steps you can take to learn the skill you want.

The last barrier, which can be a challenge for many people, is lack of social support. If people at work or at home aren't supportive of the changes you're making, developing new behaviors can be difficult. Can you think of some people who have helped you be successful in the past? You may want to enlist their support again, especially if they'll be positive about your habits.

The key to changing your habits and behaviors is starting and then moving forward. There may be some mental barriers that you have to break, but you can break them if you stay on the path. Dorothy did make it to Oz, but only because her desire to go home and to help her friends realize their dreams was strong. Together she and her friends made it. You can, too.

⌁ 9 ⌁

Chart Your Course

Dr. Seuss is famous for his children's books, but he also had a lot to say to adults. In his book *Oh, the Places You'll Go!* he wrote, "You have the brains in your head. You have feet in your shoes. You can steer yourself in any direction you choose." You may know you want to prevent diabetes, and you've probably already identified what lifestyle habits you want to develop to try to do this. But as you prepare to change and act, a plan is necessary to be successful.

One of the best ways to chart a course is by writing out your goals. There are three types of goals to write: long-term, short-term, and weekly action steps. A realistic long-term goal identifies what you hope to accomplish in the long run, such as "I will establish healthful eating and lifestyle habits to manage my weight and to prevent diabetes." Short-term goals are checkpoints along the way to assess whether you're on track toward reaching your long-term goal. A short-term goal could be "increase activity to 30 minutes per day, 6 days each week." Although it's important to know the big picture you want to achieve, it helps to focus on weekly action steps—the small steps you take to reach your long-term and short-term goals. Small changes seem more doable and add up over time. Weekly action steps are the gradual changes you make in your lifestyle habits on a daily and weekly basis to positively impact your health.

Weekly action steps work for three reasons. First, they allow you to work on one behavior change at a time. Second, they prevent you from getting overwhelmed by the larger and seemingly difficult goals you may have set. Gradual changes are easier to accept. Third, weekly action steps work because after weeks of taking these actions, you often discover that you've actually achieved some of your short-term goals and that you're well on your way to reaching your long-term goal.

To set up weekly action steps, break short-term and long-term goals down into smaller increments. Making gradual changes such as eating lunch each day, keeping low-fat foods in your desk drawer, or walking the dog a little farther a few times each week are examples of weekly action steps. When you take small steps, over time, they add up to giant leaps toward meeting your long-term goal—preventing diabetes.

Although they're called weekly action steps, it's okay to work on some for a longer time, especially if they're challenging behaviors. Then move on to a new action step. Building habits is an ongoing, step-by-step process. By starting small, being flexible, keeping goals and weekly action steps positive, and working on one behavior change at a time, you can achieve a life without diabetes.

∿ 10 ∿

Plan for Setbacks

When you were a kid, did you ever play hopscotch or Chinese jump rope or try the high jump in physical education? If you did, you might recall that in some games or sports, if you made a mistake, you needed to start at the very beginning, and with others you could start again where you left off or made the mistake.

The experience of changing any lifestyle habit can be similar to your experience with games. As we take action, moving forward in one direction, setbacks can and do happen. For instance, many people lose weight and then regain some or all of the weight they originally lost. These setbacks, which are called lapses and relapses, are a normal part of the change process. The key is acknowledging them for what they are— mistakes—learning from them, and moving forward again.

The simplest definition of a *lapse* is a slip or a mistake. If you've ever played a musical instrument, you've probably played a wrong note at some time. Playing a wrong note doesn't mean that you don't know how to play the instrument or that you're not talented. It just means that you need more practice. That's what makes a lapse different from a relapse. If you're playing the piano and you make a mistake, you can either continue playing even though the mistake was made (a lapse) or give up and quit playing for an extended period of time (relapse).

To get personal with these concepts, you might want to think about the lifestyle behaviors you're working on right now. For example, if you're regularly exercising three times a week and only exercise one time one week because of an out-of-town business trip, that's a lapse. However, if you start consistently skipping exercise, that's a relapse. You'll be returning to your

25

old habits and exposing yourself to the increased likelihood of getting diabetes.

How we respond to a lapse can determine whether the lapse will stop at a lapse or become a full-fledged relapse. A string of lapses together makes a relapse. If we lose weight and suddenly regain a few pounds, we're experiencing a lapse. We can choose to start exercising more or eating a little less to lose those few pounds, or we can choose to give up, which could cause us to regain all of the weight we lost . . . and more.

A lapse is not the end of the world; it's normal. A relapse is what you want to prevent from happening. To do this, it's important to consider the emotions, situations, or events that have the greatest potential to cause you to return to old habits. Think about it. We all react differently to internal and external cues in the environment. What emotions, situations, or events cause you to eat more, smoke more often, or skip exercising? It could be stress at work or at home, family gatherings, or feelings of loneliness.

Whatever it is, it helps to be aware of it. If you make one unhealthy choice, such as eating more than you'd like at a dinner party, it doesn't mean you have to give up all the new food habits you've been developing. Accept the mistake, acknowledge it as a learning experience, and move on. No one expects that you will be perfect at your new lifestyle behaviors, only that you will act and keep moving forward on your goal to prevent diabetes.

Unfortunately, it's easy to underestimate the importance of dealing with lapses and relapse—especially if you're on a major success run right now. But dealing with them is probably the most crucial skill needed to achieve long-term health behavior change. It's important to take time out now to envision how you'll manage lapses, or even a relapse, when they do occur. They will happen! They're a normal part of the process. Learning to handle them effectively is the trick to staying on track.

∾ 11 ∾

Celebrate Milestones

Organizations often give certificates of appreciation to volunteers. Schoolchildren make cards or gifts for their family to show their love. Employers reward valued workers with bonuses. How does such a sign of appreciation make you feel? Most likely it gives you a sense of accomplishment. It makes you feel valued as a person, and it encourages you to continue doing what you're doing.

Behavior change is no different. By rewarding ourselves for a job well done, we reinforce our new habits and move ourselves one step closer to permanent behavior change.

Anytime you set goals—long-term, short-term, or weekly action steps—it is important to develop a personal reward system. Make the reward something of personal value—a new tie, a weekend getaway, season tickets for a local sports team, a new exercise video, a manicure, or some relaxing bath oils. (Because eating habits are probably one of the areas you're working to improve, try to avoid using food as a reward.)

How often should you reward yourself? This is for you to decide. It's logical to reward yourself when you reach your short-term goals; but to stay truly motivated and to keep moving forward through the process of change, smaller successes should be noted, too. Once you've maintained new habits, such as being physically active consistently for eight weeks, you can treat yourself with something you look forward to.

One way you can track these milestones and rewards is by keeping a success journal so that you can see where you've been and how you've gotten there. Record goals you've met and how you felt about achieving the goals. Refer back to this journal often when you need extra incentive in the future.

27

Simple Changes Journal

What small changes are you ready to make *today*?

What small changes are you planning to make *this week*?

What small changes are you planning to make *this month*?

~: PART THREE :~

Manage Your Weight

At any given time, on any given day, 25 percent of men and 45 percent of women are trying to lose weight. Weight is often named as people's number one health (and beauty) concern, but up to half of all adults remain overweight. Losing weight or maintaining it as we age is a complicated issue. Yet, if we want to prevent diabetes, we need to make weight control less complicated and find a way to fit it into our daily lives.

∽ 12 ∾

The Weight-Diabetes Connection

Have you ever thought about the effects of too much body weight, other than the extra bulk? Most of us think about how it makes us look and feel and may have considered the effects on our knees, joints, and backs. Anyone with heart disease knows about the added strain that excess weight puts on the heart. What about the rest of our bodies? And what about diabetes? How does weight impact our chances of getting type 2 diabetes?

The amount of body weight you carry around does, in fact, affect your chances of getting diabetes. Excess weight makes the cells in the body resistant to insulin. Your body still makes insulin, but added weight prevents your body from using it the way it should. For this reason, body weight has a definite connection to whether you'll get diabetes. If you're heavy, you're more likely to get diabetes. If you're at a healthy weight—and stay there—you're less likely to get this disease.

So managing your weight is a given. If you think you're currently overweight, you can help prevent diabetes by shedding some pounds. Lowering body weight by as little as 5 to 10 percent (10 to 20 pounds if you weigh 200 pounds) can improve your odds against getting diabetes. If you consider yourself to be at a healthy weight right now, remember that the average person gains 20 pounds between the ages of 25 and 55, so you're not necessarily off the hook. Your goal is to maintain your current healthy weight.

The good news is that up to half of all cases of type 2 diabetes could be prevented if people achieved and maintained healthy body weights. And because diabetes isn't curable, prevention is key for living into the golden years without serious health problems.

31

✌ 13 ✌

Weight Gain Doesn't Happen Overnight

Computer games. Video games. Remote controls. Self-propelled lawn mowers. Clothes washers and dryers. Elevators. Garage door openers. We don't think twice about using these devices to make our lives easier. But, unfortunately, their use isn't doing anything to benefit our health. Our bodies were not designed for inactivity, yet we get less and less activity in our daily lives thanks to all these technological advances. In fact, 24 percent of us lead completely inactive lives, and only one out of five gets the recommended level of exercise. Limited daily activity combined with only occasional bouts of structured exercise translates into burning fewer calories, which can in turn lead to weight gain. And being overweight is the one factor most likely to increase our chances of getting type 2 diabetes.

Although lack of activity does contribute to being overweight, it is not the only factor. What we eat is equally important. Half of the average food budget is spent on food prepared and/or eaten outside the home—in restaurants, at work cafeterias, in cars after cruising through the drive-through of the local fast-food establishment, and after a quick call to the nearest pizza delivery house. These places don't always offer the healthiest food choices, or if they do, we don't order them. Although the amount of fat we eat has dropped in the past decade, the average person now weighs more. How did this happen? Probably because we get more calories than we did 10 years ago, even though fewer of them come from fat.

The third factor that helps decide whether we'll be overweight is our genetic blueprint. Are your grandparents overweight? Your parents? Your brothers and sisters? If so, you're more likely to be overweight. Much of the research on the genetic component of obesity was done on twins who were separated at birth. Even though they were raised in different environments, most sets of twins will have similar body weights as adults—both being thin, both being average weight, or both being overweight. Today, researchers are trying to identify the gene or the group of genes that lends a hand in causing obesity, and one day there may be an answer.

The reality is that extra pounds do not sneak up on you overnight. The typical person gradually gains 20 pounds between the ages of 25 and 55, and these three factors—activity, eating habits, and genetics—are what influence the gain. So if you want to live longer, be healthier, and prevent diabetes, make these factors work for you, not against you. If you're at a healthy weight now, do what it takes to stay there. If you're overweight, examine your lifestyle habits and consider what changes you can make to shed some pounds.

~: 14 :~

Find Your Motivation

For many of us, it's not a news flash that we weigh too much. Maybe we're secure enough in our lives that the paunch of middle age doesn't bother us. Or maybe we've been overweight for all of our adult years and have learned to live with it. Our weight could have yo-yoed so much over the years that we're sure there's no real solution to losing weight and keeping it off. Some women are too busy to deal with the 20 extra pounds three pregnancies have left behind. We don't do anything about extra weight because the threat of diabetes doesn't seem real enough.

So what about you? Are you worried enough about diabetes to try to shed those extra pounds? Have you given any thought to what it will take to motivate you to examine and change your habits? What barriers are stopping you from taking action today, right this minute, in fact?

It is okay if improved health and diabetes prevention aren't your primary motivation for losing weight. There can be many other personal benefits to getting to a lower number on the scale. What about appearance? Feeling better? Looking sexier? Fitting into a smaller size? Creating a body as buff as the 25-year-old who lives next door? Feeling muscles in your arms and legs that you never knew existed? Keeping up with your kids as they in-line skate through the neighborhood?

One way to figure out what will motivate you to make changes in your lifestyle is to think of all the benefits you'll personally gain when you lose weight. No matter how silly or selfish they may seem, write down ten benefits in a journal or a notebook or on a stray piece of paper. Then force yourself to come up with ten more benefits—it's often the second ten that are the real reasons you want to lose weight. In these you may find the real motivation for making a conscientious effort to manage your weight.

Putting all this into writing can make you see up front what you could gain if you started taking steps to manage your weight. Then once you're on the path toward a healthier lifestyle, this list will motivate you, reenergize you, and get you through the rough spots.

What Does a Healthy Weight
Look Like, Anyway?

A news television program once did an episode on linemen in the National Football League (NFL) and how dramatically their weights have increased over the past twenty years. Many of them tip the scales at well over 300 pounds. Yet today's fashion models have brought back the idea that the thinner you are, the better. So which direction is right? How do you decide if you're at a healthy weight? If you're not, how many pounds do you need to lose to prevent diabetes?

Right now, the best tool to use in deciding if your current weight is healthy is the BMI—*body mass index*. Essentially, the BMI is a math formula that relates to body fat, and it is better at predicting the risk of disease than body weight alone. If you want to know your BMI, multiply your weight in pounds by 700 and divide the product by your height in inches squared.

$$\text{BMI} = \frac{\text{weight} \times 700}{\text{height} \times \text{height}}$$

If you weigh 200 pounds and are 5 feet 7 inches tall, for example, your BMI would be 31 (200×700 divided by 67×67, or $140,000 \div 4,489$). If the result is a number between 19 and 25, you're at a healthy weight and your goal should be to maintain this weight as you age. A number of 27 or higher is an indication that you are overweight and puts you at higher risk for many diseases, including diabetes.

This same equation can be used to determine a healthy weight and an appropriate weight-loss goal. If your BMI is above the recommended 25, calculate the weight at which you would need to be to have a BMI of 25 ($25 \times$ height [in inches] $\times$ height divided by 700). Then subtract your answer from your current weight to find your weight-loss goal. When looking at the weight that would get your BMI to 25, there are several things you need to consider: Does the number seem realistic? Is it a weight you've been able to maintain as an adult before? Do you think you could maintain this weight without starving yourself or exercising excessively?

Once you've taken all these factors into account, you can decide if this is the right target weight for you. If you're not comfortable with it and already had a figure in mind, you can use that, assuming it's a realistic goal. If, for example, you are a woman in your midfifties and have had five children, it's probably not realistic to aim for the same weight you were when you got married. You could just calculate 5 or 10 percent of your current weight and use this as your weight-loss goal. Afterall, this change can be enough to prevent diabetes. Whatever you decide to use as a weight-loss goal—the number from the BMI chart, 10 percent of your current body weight, or another number—don't let the goal overwhelm you to the point that you don't take action.

If your goal is a high number, say over 50 or 75 pounds, you should consider using it as a long-term goal, something to be accomplished over the next three to five years. Breaking it down into manageable steps can work, aiming to lose 20 pounds the first year, to maintain this loss for six months, and then to tackle the next 20 pounds. Whatever your goal, weight loss of one-half to one pound per week is a realistic expectation and sets you on a path to finding your own healthy weight.

~: 16 ~

Factor in Body Shape
to Your Health Equation

We all know that fruit is a healthy food choice. But have you ever given much thought to the lesson that fruit can teach about your chances of developing certain diseases like diabetes?

There's more to deciding if our weight is healthy than looking at our BMI. We should also look at where that weight is carried. This is where fruit comes in—more specifically, apples and pears. But we're not really talking fruit here, we're talking body shape. Apple-shaped people—those who carry excess weight at their waists—are more likely to get many diseases, including type 2 diabetes. Pear-shaped people—those who carry excess weight around the hips—are less likely to get these same diseases.

But how can you tell if you're an apple or a pear? Simple. You just need to get out the tape measure, measure the inches around your waist, and then the inches around the widest portion of your hips. The waist measurement is then divided by the hip measurement. This handy test is called the *waist-to-hip ratio*. If your waist number is higher than your hip number, you are an apple. If the hip number is higher, you are a pear.

WAIST-TO-HIP RATIO		Pear	Apple
Waist	38	28	44
Hip	38	35	40
Waist-to-Hip Ratio	1.0	0.8	1.1

Men with a waist-to-hip ratio greater than 1.0 are at greater risk for high blood pressure, heart disease, and diabetes. For women, higher risk starts at a ratio of 0.8.

So even though apples and pears may be just about equal from a nutritional standpoint, apple and pear body shapes definitely are not equal when it comes to developing diabetes and other diseases. Your weight may be just right for you, but where you carry that weight may be putting you at higher risk for diabetes. Your body shape is one more factor to consider in determining what action you personally need to take to prevent diabetes.

~ 17 ~

Inch Your Way to Success

So what is weight anyway? What does that number on the scale really tell you? You could see three people who all weigh the exact same amount, but whose bodies look totally different. One could be a short athlete. One could be tall and thin. One could be pregnant. A 300-pound couch potato would look nothing like one of those linemen from the National Football League. Yes, most of them weigh *over* 300 pounds, but many have a very low percentage of body fat. They have masses of muscle developed by working out several hours each day.

The point is that we give too much weight to that number on the scale when we're trying to lose weight. We've all been there before—we have a great week, really watching what we're eating and exercising on three days. On Saturday, we hop on the scale and find that we've lost only one-fourth of a pound. We get discouraged and wonder if it's even worth the effort.

We all need to keep in mind that weight can fluctuate on a weekly basis for a variety of reasons—how much fluids we've had to drink, where a woman is in her menstrual cycle, and so forth. On a long-term basis, weight may not go down as quickly as we'd like for the simple reason that muscle weighs more than fat. By getting active, we're building muscle and burning calories. As we combine healthier eating with this activity, we're losing even more fat. So our weight may not drop dramatically. Yet, this is a good thing. We want to lose fat and gain muscle. Although some of us can't resist using a scale as a measurement of our progress, we shouldn't weigh ourselves more than once a week, and we need to keep in mind why the number change may be small.

But the scale is only one way to measure success. Another way to look at the real strides you're making toward a healthier life is to use the tape measure one more time. If you think it would be useful to you, measure various parts of your body either on your own or with the help of a supportive friend or family member (or even an employee at your health club). The most common measurements done include the upper arm, neck, chest, waist, hips, and thighs. It can be helpful to keep a record of the numbers in a notebook or other convenient place and to repeat the process every two months or so.

As you initially lose weight and start to tone up, you'll find the inches decreasing in almost every area. But you need to be forewarned that if you exercise consistently, some numbers, such as your arms and chest, may start to increase again. This is a good thing. It means you're gaining muscle.

By using the tape you'll be pleasantly surprised with the results and decrease your dependence on the scale. You'll realize you've found a new measure of success—inches.

~: 18 :~

Skip the Pills—for Now

We live in a world of pill-popping. We get a headache, we take a pill. We sense a cold coming on, and we try to prevent it with the latest cold remedy. We haven't been eating many fruits or vegetables lately, so out come the supplements. Our stomach gets a little upset, and another pill comes to the rescue. No wonder we think that we can solve being overweight with a pill.

Much research is, in fact, being done on drugs that help people lose weight. And there may be a role for these drugs for those of us who, despite building healthful lifestyle habits, can't lose weight because of our genes. We might eat low fat foods, limit portion sizes, and exercise several days of the week and still be overweight. Medications—combined with a healthy lifestyle—may be our answer to successful weight loss.

But, unfortunately, the perfect medication hasn't arrived yet. Many drugs would require that you take them for the rest of your life to keep weight off. Yet the effects of taking these drugs for years and decades hasn't been studied. Some of the obesity drugs developed recently had to be pulled off the market because of serious negative side effects (almost all medications have some side effects). You should weigh the pros and cons of taking any medication with a health care provider.

But what about those over-the-counter options like appetite suppressants and liquid diets? Unfortunately, few of them have been proven to really cause weight loss. And, unlike prescibed obesity medications, they don't deal with genetics—the issue that may be preventing you from reaching your goal weight. Furthermore, no medications help you change your habits—whether it's eating for emotional reasons rather than for hunger, having a hard time finding the motivation to exercise regularly, or understanding where the fat really is in the foods you eat.

So, although medications do provide some answers today and definite hope for the future, make sure you take *all* the steps you can to manage your weight and prevent diabetes. Talk to your doctor about currently available obesity medications and whether they're right for you. But at the same time, it's important to look at your lifestyle and where you can make positive changes. No medication will work if you're not changing your habits at the same time.

~: 19 :~

Binge Eating May Be Doing You In

E ven though you've been very focused all week on healthful eating and getting active, do you find yourself one night going on a binge, eating whatever happens to be around? When this happens, do you taste the flavor of the food? Are you conscious of what foods you're eating? Or do you feel a total loss of control over the eating occasion? Later on, do you feel guilty or depressed?

This can be a frustrating experience for all of us, especially when we felt we were finally starting to get a handle on building positive lifestyle habits and managing our weight. These periodic food cravings that get out of hand can sabotage our efforts to improve our health.

If this is a problem for you, you're not alone. Up to a third of people who are overweight struggle with binge eating. For most people, binges happen three to five times a week, and usually consist of high fat foods. This behavior is such a problem and so prevalent that it's actually been diagnosed by medical professionals and given a name—Binge Eating Disorder. Bear in mind, however, that there's a difference between a periodic binge (who doesn't eat a few too many when making chocolate chip cookies?) and the disorder. If binges happen several times a week and are out of control, then you probably have Binge Eating Disorder.

If you even suspect you may have this disorder, you should seek help. Why? Because positive lifestyle changes that you make can be counteracted by binge eating. In fact, if you've tried to lose weight in the past without success, Binge Eating Disorder could have been the reason. So you need to address this disorder separately from your efforts to lose weight.

The two professionals to seek out for help with Binge Eating Disorder are a licensed therapist who specializes in eating disorders and a registered dietitian. They can help get the binges under control. During this period in counseling, you won't be focusing specifically on losing weight. The focus is on the issues that can trigger the binges. Once you're better able to manage the binging, you can look toward real success with managing weight.

SIMPLE CHANGES JOURNAL

What small changes can you make *today* to manage your weight?

What small changes can you make *this week* to manage your weight?

What small changes can you make *this month* to manage your weight?

∾ PART FOUR ∾

Real Nutrition for Real People

You've seen the Food Guide Pyramid and all it's variations. You've read all the new diet books that are just recycles of those written 25 years ago. You constantly are bombarded with new low fat, no fat, and reduced fat products on supermarket shelves. It's information overload, that's what it is. How do you make sense out of all this nutrition chaos? To prevent diabetes and to lose weight, you don't want a high-tech system. You just want actions you can take in the areas of nutrition that really matter for better health.

～ 20 ～

Follow the 80/20 Rule

Have you ever told yourself that you'll go on a *diet* for the next three months to lose 10 pounds, and then after that three month period, you find yourself returning to your old eating and lifestyle habits? Or if you plan to start a *diet* on Monday, do you eat all your favorite foods over the weekend? For most of us *diet* indicates a beginning and an end, and that is exactly why you should throw the word *diet* out of your vocabulary. Replace *diet* with a new phrase—*consistent eating plan*. This is the real key to lifelong management of weight. The goal is to make changes in your eating habits that you can live with and maintain on a regular basis. To accomplish this level of consistency, you need the 80/20 Rule: If 80 percent of the time you make healthful food choices, the other 20 percent can fall through the cracks without adversely affecting your health.

The trick with this rule is focusing on the 80 percent days. Your food choices on these days need to be really nutritious—low fat meals, plenty of fruits and vegetables, and proper-sized portions of food. This rule means that you will pass by the candy dish on your co-worker's desk most of the time, choose the side salad instead of French fries at a fast-food restaurant, and make snack time fruit time. The 20 percent days are holidays, vacations, and special occasions. If you're careful on the 80 percent days, then when the 20 percent days come along, you can truly enjoy the eating occasion without feeling guilty and know that you're still on track for diabetes prevention and weight management.

The 80/20 Rule—consider making it your motto for a lifetime of consistent, healthful eating habits.

❧ 21 ❧

The Skinny on Fat

Fat—it's the issue that's been at the forefront of everything we've read and heard about in nutrition for the past 10 years. And, truth be told, that's where it should be, especially because we're interested in preventing diabetes and managing our weight. The goal for each of us is to get less than 30 percent of each day's calories from fat (65 grams of fat or less, for the average person), but most of us are still getting more than that. Even though this message is repeated time and time again, it seems as if many of us haven't heard it yet.

How can you eat so that your fat intake is less than 65 grams per day? Well, that depends on your personality. Anytime you make changes in your habits, it's important to do it in a way that fits your style. This is especially true when it comes to the food choices you make. Because you have to eat food to survive and because you eat several times every day, it's essential that your method for building healthier eating habits suits your personal style.

Suppose you're a spontaneous person who works best under pressure. Planning out low fat meals two weeks in advance will never work for you. But you might find long-term success at building low fat eating habits by gathering some information to have handy for quick meal solutions. What kind of information? For starters, the most healthful options at local fast-food and take-out restaurants, the best tasting low fat frozen dinners, and the brands of your favorite foods that are the lowest in fat. Using this information to make simple changes on a daily basis can significantly lower the amount of fat you eat over time.

For those who are analytical planners, a more intensive approach to low fat eating habits might be the way to go. This can include a *fat budget;* that is, you determine the right number of fat grams to have each day, and then you track how much fat you get to make sure you stay within your budget. To find your starting fat budget, you may want to write down everything you eat for three days. Then figure out the total calories, and divide by three to find your average calories. If your goal is to lose weight, subtract 250 to 500 calories from this number. Take this new number, multipy it by 0.3, and divide that answer by 9. This is your starting fat budget.

Try staying within this budget for a few days. If you find it a challenge to consistently keep your fat grams this low, you've found the right starting point for you. If, on the other hand, it's easy for you to stay below this fat budget, drop 5 to 10 grams off your budget, and use this as your daily goal.

No matter what your style, there's flexibility in how you cut back on fat. In fact, it's almost impossible to eat low fat every single day. Business lunches and dinner with friends on the weekend might affect the fat grams you get on any one particular day. It's the weekly average that counts. If over a week's time, the average amount of fat you eat is lower, you're on track for managing your weight. You can use this to your benefit, too. If you know you're heading to a sporting event on Friday night and will probably eat a meal that is higher than usual in fat, you can cut back 5 to 10 fat grams each day during the week. Then you'll be able to enjoy your night out knowing you've planned for it.

When it comes to limiting your fat intake, there are lots of ways to do it—many more than the two options mentioned here. The point is that whatever method you choose, it needs to fit your personality and lifestyle.

❧ 22 ❧

Make Your Goal
Consistent Eating Habits

We've all been raised in a society that believes if a little is good, more must be better—money, vitamins, you name it. So, if dropping to 25 percent or 30 percent of calories from fat in eating habits is good, wouldn't lower be even better? Isn't no fat the ultimate goal? While we've been programmed to believe this, it's not the mentality we need for weight management to prevent diabetes.

The real secret to finding long-term success in healthy behaviors is building habits you can live with for the rest of your life. Consistency, remember? Although 10 percent of calories from fat sounds great—the pounds will just fall off, diabetes wouldn't even think of striking you—you need to ask yourself if it's a habit you can maintain forever. Odds are, it isn't. Besides, the body does need some fat. And this doesn't say anything about your will power or lack of it. It's just reality. Maintaining a very low fat or no fat eating plan indefinitely is an almost impossible feat for anyone. So the best idea is to start at 30 percent of calories from fat and drop this number lower (but not below 20 percent of calories from fat) as you feel ready. Low fat eating is a habit you want not just for three weeks or three months but for the rest of your life.

The other reality to consider when thinking about reducing fat is that gradual changes are better and easier than drastic changes. You've lived with your current habits for a long time. It takes little steps, added up over time, to make big changes in these habits. So again, starting at 30 percent of calories from fat is the right thing to do. Then you can cut back a few fat grams in two weeks. Then in a month you cut back a few more fat grams. Then a few more come spring. Soon you'll find yourself with a much lower fat intake. And it if it takes a year or two to get to your goal, it's okay. All along, you're making improvements, you're headed in the right direction, and you're staying on track.

In the end, the important question to ask yourself is not "How low can I go?" but "How long can I keep it up?" That's the real challenge.

∽ 23 ∾

The Calorie Comeback

We call it the "No Fat Cookie Diet." Several years ago, when all the low and no fat foods hit the grocery store shelves, we went crazy. Finally, there were great tasting, no-guilt foods available that satisfied our craving for the sweet stuff. So we ate cookies and brownies, and made cakes from the low fat mixes, and indulged without an ounce of guilt. After all, they were fat free. We could eat all we want, right?

We all found out soon enough that these products weren't really harmless. True, they have very little fat, but they still have *calories*. Oh yes, calories! Even though food manufacturers had found a way to take out all the fat, they hadn't really made the calorie counts any lower than their traditional high fat counterparts. How come? When they took the fat out, they had to replace it with something, and in many cases, that something was sugar. So fat came down, but calories didn't. Overall, we were eating less fat, but we were not losing weight because we were getting more calories. And excess weight increases the odds of getting diabetes.

One of the biggest reasons that building low fat eating habits can help with weight management is that you cut down on the most calorie-dense types of foods there are—fats. Ounce for ounce, fat has more calories than do carbohydrates (bread, cereal, pasta, fruits, potatoes, corn), protein (lean meats), and alcohol. By cutting down on fat, you automatically get fewer calories than you used to get. Less fat and fewer calories add up to weight loss. This equation works unless you continue to indulge on all the low and no fat treats available.

That's why the calorie has made a comeback. Today, we're all tuning into calories as well as fat grams. This doesn't mean you need to track your daily calories as well as fat (you want to keep this simple, right?), but it does mean that the amounts of low and no fat foods you eat matter. After all, products with just one gram of fat aren't sold with a license to eat as many as you want. If you used to eat two regular cookies, eat two low fat cookies instead. If you used to make cakes only on special occasions, do the same. Just make the low fat version now. By taking steps like these, you can all keep calories in check while focusing on fat. But by all means if tracking both fat grams and calories is the method that works for you, do so. It's your personal plan for weight management and diabetes prevention.

✌ 24 ✍

No Room for Supersizing

Have you noticed that we live in an era of supersizing? Consider the 32-ounce single serving of soda, the supersizing of fast-food meals for a mere fifty cents added to the regular price, huge muffins and cinnamon buns in coffee shops, warehouse grocery stores (that only sell in bulk) in every city. How are you to manage your weight in this kind of eating environment?

Weight management isn't easy with all this supersizing going on, but it isn't impossible either. It is true that you can eat anything you want, but weight management is about how much of each food you eat and how often you eat. It's simply a matter of taking a realistic look at portion sizes of the foods you eat and of knowing which food portions to watch more closely.

You already have some tools to use to get familiar with the portions of food you eat—food labels, measuring cups, and the plates, bowls, glasses and cups you use regularly at home. If you want to use food labels to help you manage your portions of food, look at the areas of the Nutrition Facts panel marked "Serving Size" and "Servings per Container." The serving size tells you the specific amount of that food on which the nutrition information, including the fat grams, is based. Depending on the food, the serving size could be given in ounces (meat), fractions of a cup (vegetables, ice cream, cereal), slices (bread, packaged cheese), and so on.

To find the correct portion size of, for example, breakfast cereal, look at the nutrition panel on the box. The serving size might be ¾ cup or 1 cup. You can simply fill a measuring cup with the proper amount of the food to see what one portion looks like. Or you can pour your usual serving of cereal into your bowl, then pour that into a measuring cup, and compare the amount with the standard serving size. If you find that you usually eat two portions of cereal for breakfast, that's fine, but at least now you know how much your typical portion amounts to.

Servings per container are useful on canned or frozen prepared products. If a can of soup says it serves two and you usually eat the whole can by yourself, multiply the fat grams by two to know the real debit against your fat budget.

The second tool for portion control is your dishes. It is very helpful for a week or two to measure out how much food you put into the plates, bowls, glasses, and cups you use frequently. Once you know the amounts that fit into your different dishes, you'll be able to more accurately gauge the amounts of food you're eating, the fat grams in these foods, and the foods for which you might need to decrease your portion size. It's a good idea, too, every so often to remeasure so your eye doesn't lose its version of the portion sizes that fit into your dishes.

It's obvious that you need to monitor portion sizes in order to manage weight. But do you need to check portions of everything you eat? Actually, you don't need to track everything. Plain fruits (but not juice) and vegetables, for example, are foods that are so good for you that you can never really get too much of them, so you shouldn't worry about limiting your portions. Plain pasta, rice, and other similar products can also be watched less closely, again because they're so low in fat. The items you want to monitor closely include high fat items like regular salad dressings, butter, and mayonnaise; creamy sauces; many meats; cheeses; snack items like chips; and dessert items like cakes, cookies, and ice creams.

The key point to remember, though, is that this doesn't give you a license to eat large quantities of low fat foods. Listen to your body, let it tell you how hungry you are, and eat only the amount needed to satisfy that hunger. If you're not losing weight or find you're having a tough time maintaining your weight, it doesn't necessarily mean that the foods you choose need to change. It might be that you're getting too much food and, in the end, too many calories. If you read food labels and measure foods, you can manage your portions.

∽ 25 ∼

Assess Your Hunger

Do you ever find yourself heading to the cafeteria for lunch just because it's noon—even if you're not really hungry? Do you seek comfort in ice cream after an argument with a significant other? Or are you the type of person who can be so engrossed in a project that you don't realize you missed both breakfast and lunch and now feel as if you're about to faint?

Consider these scenarios and you'll begin to realize that we all eat for different reasons and for distinct reasons at different times. Many of us have lost sight of the real reason to eat—hunger. The sensation of hunger is the signal that our bodies need food—the fuel they use to run efficiently. In today's society where all social situations and many business occasions revolve around food, we can find it difficult to stay in tune with our real need for food. We need to reacquaint ourselves with hunger, especially if we're concerned about managing our weight to prevent diabetes.

The first step in getting to know your personal hunger feeling is to understand the difference between physical hunger and emotional hunger. If you're truly physically hungry, your body will tell you through such signals as a rumbling stomach, difficulty concentrating, light-headedness, a headache, or even the feeling that you're going to faint. Your hunger signal can be different from that of the next person, but the message is essentially the same: "I need food and I need it now."

Emotional hunger, on the other hand, is looking for food in response to emotions—boredom, depression, frustration, anger, or happiness. You have so much pent up emotion that you don't know what to do with it or don't allow yourself to feel the emotion, so you eat in response to it, with the hope that

58

food will soothe it or stuff it down. Obviously, this has nothing to do with *hunger*, a real physical need for food.

Are you unsure of whether you're eating in response to physical hunger or emotional hunger? Join the club. Many of us have lost touch with our sense of hunger. But we can find it again.

If you want to determine whether you're eating to fuel your body, you can use this simple tool: The next time you're reaching for a snack or some candy, ordering take-out food, or thinking about making a meal, stop yourself for one minute. Take just one minute to assess your current hunger-meter reading by asking yourself the following questions: What physical signs of hunger do I have? On a scale of 1 to 10 (with 1 being not hungry and 10 being very hungry), how hungry am I? A 2 indicates a need for a snack. A 5 might be satisifed by a light lunch. If it's a 9, a full meal is called for.

If you realize that you don't have any of the physical signs of hunger, you may be eating for emotional reasons. Finding something else to do to release the emotion, such as exercising, journaling, talking it out with someone, or confronting the other person involved, can feed this emotional hunger. If you do have physical signs of hunger, well then eat, and enjoy the eating occasion. You really are eating to fuel your body's needs.

It's a good idea to assess your hunger again on the 1 to 10 scale halfway through a meal or snack. To be efficient at managing your weight and controlling your portions of food, it's best to stop eating when you're feeling about 80 percent full. Because it takes some time for the "full" signal to travel from your stomach to your brain, stopping at 80 percent full will result in a 100 percent full feeling 20 minutes after eating. For managing weight and preventing diabetes, the trick is using your hunger meter to your advantage.

∿ 26 ∿

The Clean Plate Club

"Don't leave food on your plate when there are starving kids in Africa." "Finish everything on your plate or else there's no dessert for you." Did you grow up hearing messages like these? Many of us did. And if you did, it can be more than a little difficult to stop eating when you're full. We've been programmed to believe these messages, making it very difficult for us to leave food on our plates even when we're no longer hungry. This can make managing weight more of a struggle.

The trick is to reprogram your thoughts. Some suggestions on how to cancel a membership in the Clean Plate Club include:

- Think rationally. Leaving food on your plate doesn't directly affect starving people in other parts of the world.

- Practice leaving small amounts of food on your plate. Leaving one or two bites at every meal helps you get used to doing it.

- If you initially feel guilty leaving food on your plate, make donations to hunger organizations that really do help the fight against hunger and starvation.

- Take small portions at the beginning of a meal. After eating this amount, assess your hunger. If you're still hungry, take another small portion.

- As soon as you're finished eating, remove the plate from your sight. This will prevent the leftover bites from tempting you.

- At a restaurant (where portions are almost always larger than necessary to satisfy your hunger), ask for the plate to be cleared as soon as you hit 80 percent full. If enough of your meal remains, ask for a "doggie" bag.

❖ 27 ❖

Take a Lesson from a Child and Eat Intuitively

Overeaters Anonymous tells its clients to completely avoid temptation foods—those foods that send them into an overeating frenzy. They tell their members to never again eat those foods. Some diet gurus say we should never eat individual foods that have more than 30 percent of their calories from fat—no butter, margarine, or oil ever again; no bacon; no eggs; no potato chips; no doughnuts or sweets. For years, health professionals have said, "No red meat. It's bad for you. It will cause heart disease. Stay away from it."

If you look at these statements objectively, do any of them make sense? The reality is that we have to eat. We need food to fuel our bodies, so we can perform our everyday activities. And if we do what these messages tell us—to avoid certain "bad" foods—we're only setting ourselves up for failure out of desperation. It's human nature to *crave* what we can't have. So what can we do? Eat intuitively.

But what does that mean? If you have young children of your own or in your extended group of family or friends, watch them closely when it comes to their eating habits. Infants and toddlers have an innate sense about food if no one interferes with it. They eat when they're hungry. They stop when they're full. They don't follow a clock that tells them to eat lunch at noon and dinner at six. They listen to their bodies. More importantly, if they're given free access to food, young children eat what they're hungry for and what their bodies need. And they enjoy it—the food, the eating occasion, the whole experience.

You can learn to act more like children—at least when it comes to your eating habits. You've already worked on getting in touch with your hunger, but it's also important to give yourself permission to eat any and all foods. Food in and of itself isn't bad. It's what you do with food that can be less than good. The first step is to allow any and all foods into your kitchen. If you love chocolate, you should have chocolate. If it's salty snacks you crave, you can have them. Giving yourself permission to eat the foods you really love can dramatically change your relationship with food.

The trick in this is to listen to your body. What is it that you're really craving? If the answer is a doughnut, but you tell yourself you can't have a doughnut and have toast instead, you're setting yourself up for a craving that will last throughout the day. You'll try to fill that craving with so many different things that you'll consume more calories and fat grams than if you just had eaten the one doughnut! So if you're hungry for a doughnut, have a doughnut, but stop at just one. You can eat anything you want as long as you wait until you're physically hungry and stop when you're satisfied. Besides, most often it's that first taste, the first few bites that fill the need and give you a feeling of satisfaction.

Every time you're hungry, tune into your body, and let it tell you what it needs. And enjoy the eating experience. After all, a big part of eating is enjoying it—the aroma, the flavor and texture, and the good memories certain foods may bring. By truly listening to your body, you'll find that most often you'll be hungry for foods that are good for you—fruits, vegetables, milk, yogurt, breads, pastas, and lean meats. And by eating what you're hungry for, you'll be satisfied and not on a continual hunt for something to soothe a craving.

~: 28 ~

Find Your Food Triggers

Have you ever noticed that in today's society we've been pro-grammed to eat for many reasons other than hunger? We eat at noon because that's lunchtime. Many married people eat two big meals on holidays because they have to visit both sides of the family. Spectators eat at a football game because everyone does. After a confrontation at work, you may eat a candy bar to deal with the frustration.

The reality is that we're not necessarily physically hungry when we eat in situations like these. So why are we eating? Often we aren't aware of the reason why we eat or overeat. It's almost subconscious. We just do it.

So what can you do about this subconscious eating, espe-cially when it isn't doing anything for your weight management efforts? Begin by looking at what happens before the eating actually begins. What is it that triggered you to think about eat-ing? You'll probably find that you are turning to food in response to one or more of these five triggers: sensory cues, spe-cial events, activities, people, or emotions.

Eating in response to the sight or the smell of food usually indicates that the overeating is triggered by *sensory cues*. Fresh pastries in the window of a bakery lure you inside. Food sitting on the countertop calls to you even though you had dinner an hour ago. Food commercials make your mouth water and send you to the kitchen in search of a snack.

If you're at a potluck dinner, do you find you have to try everything? Do you overindulge on all the once-a-year foods on Thanksgiving? Do you enjoy vacation partially because it's an opportunity to try new tastes and flavors? If this sounds like you, you're probably someone who responds to *special events* triggers.

Those of us who respond to *activity* triggers associate food with activities like sporting events, movies, and television watching. Popcorn at the movies, a bag of chips during Thursday night sitcoms, or a full play-by-play about the snacks at a Super Bowl party are all part of the routine here.

Do you have an eating friend—someone you can count on when you're really in the mood for junk food? If so, you may be someone who responds to *people* triggers. You tend to plan social activities and get togethers around eating events. Happy hour wouldn't be nearly as happy without the fabulous appetizers, right?

Emotional triggers affect a lot of people. An argument with a boss, feeling lonely on the weekends, anxiety about waiting to hear about a promotion, or joy over the birth of a grandchild can all cause us to eat or to overeat.

After considering these different triggers, you may have the answer for why, where, and how you eat when you're not physically hungry. But knowing what sends you in search of food is only the first step. It's also important to figure out how to change these behaviors. Unfortunately just one trick doesn't work for everyone or for all triggers. If you think they'll be useful to you, try some of the following ideas for dealing with your triggers in ways that don't involve eating.

- *Sensory triggers.* Try keeping tempting foods in opaque containers (out of sight, out of mind). Channel surf during television commercials, never staying too long on one that shows food. Purchase healthful options like fresh-baked bread at a bakery. Change driving routes to avoid fast-food restaurants that tempt you.

- *Special event triggers.* Use the smallest plate available at a buffet or a potluck dinner. Choose a health-oriented vacation instead of a 12-meal-a-day cruise. Host a party so you can control the menu. Look for magazine and newspaper articles that tell you how to make low fat versions of holiday dishes.

- *Activity triggers.* Keep your hands busy while watching television—crocheting, knitting, crossword puzzles, or any other hobby will work. Look for healthful snack options—pretzels, frozen yogurt, grilled chicken sandwiches—that are now offered at many sports facilities. Time your arrival at the movies so you don't have time to get munchies.

- *People triggers.* Think of all the activities you can do with your favorite people that don't involve food—in-line skating, golfing, bowling, window shopping at the mall, a trip to the local zoo. Also think about turning your eating friends into healthful habit friends. You might be surprised at how interested they are in making this change, too.

- *Emotional triggers.* Confront the co-worker with whom you argued and settle your differences. Exercise to release all the stress. Sit down with a tall glass of icewater and listen to a relaxation tape. Call a friend who likes to listen. Comfort yourself by buying a good paperback instead of a sundae.

You may not have realized the effect these triggers have on you, but they could have been stopping you from eating more healthfully and losing weight. Managing them will prevent them from tripping you up.

∽ 29 ∾

Strive for Five

No, it's not the new local running race, the latest Internet site, or a hot new video game. It's a simple goal that can have a big impact on your health.

So what does it mean? "Strive for five" encourages all of us to eat five servings of fruits and vegetables every day. Why? The biggest reason is that if we truly strive for five, we'll find that we're not hungry for all the extra snacky stuff that has calories and fat but not many other nutrients. If we fill up on fruits and vegetables, we'll get lots of good things like fiber and vitamins. The end result will be fewer fat grams, fewer calories, and help with losing weight. Any weight loss improves our odds against getting diabetes. Wow; all that from getting five!

So what counts as a part of five a day? Anything and everything we consider a fruit or a vegetable. Juice counts. Dried fruits like raisins count. And it doesn't have to be fresh produce. Frozen and canned fruits and vegetables count, too, and they can be just as nutritious as fresh produce.

For many of us the most confusing point about strive for five is that it's five servings, not five separate fruits and vegetables each day. But what counts as a serving? In general, one serving is equal to a medium-sized fruit or vegetable, one-half cup of juice or a cooked vegetable, or one cup of raw fruits or vegetables (strawberry or carrot chunks, for example). So if your lunch is a salad that has two cups of romaine lettuce plus sliced tomatoes, onions, and grated carrots, you've gotten in three of your five for the day.

When you're just getting started with strive for five, it takes a conscious effort to include fruits and vegetables throughout the day. The following tips can help you get started.

STRIVE FOR FIVE TIPS

- Add fruit to your cereal in the morning.
- Have a glass of juice as a midmorning snack.
- Grab fruit that's ready to eat, like bananas and apples, to have in the car or on the bus ride to work.
- Keep fruits and vegetables visible. Instead of storing them in a refrigerator drawer, arrange them on the kitchen counters or table.
- After a grocery shopping trip, cut up celery, cauliflower, and broccoli to have for munching on throughout the week.
- Buy the packaged baby carrots as a handy snack or sandwich side dish.
- Have a large baked potato as a meal in itself. Top with chives and fat free sour cream or plain yogurt instead of butter and regular sour cream.
- Purchase frozen and canned vegetables for later in the week when the fresh stuff is all gone.
- Mix frozen peas, shredded carrots, onions, and rutabagas into meat loaves, chili, and casseroles.
- Add sprouts, sliced tomatoes and cucumbers, lettuce, and onions to sandwiches.

SIMPLE CHANGES JOURNAL

What small changes can you make *today* to improve your eating habits?

What small changes can you make *this week* to improve your eating habits?

What small changes can you make *this month* to improve your eating habits?

✌: PART FIVE ∼

Get Moving,
Get Fit

Modern technology makes our lives easier, but that doesn't mean it makes our lives healthier. More than 60 percent of us lead inactive lifestyles, and lack of activity is one of the major lifestyle habits increasing our chances of developing diabetes. We all think it takes running marathons to improve our health, but the reality is that it doesn't take that much exercise to make a difference. Small amounts of day-to-day activity and consistent amounts of exercise will benefit your health.

⌁ 30 ⌁

The Benefits of an Active Lifestyle

Each year Americans spend billions of dollars on nutritional supplements, searching for that magic pill or potion that can help them lose weight, become more fit, stay healthy, or look or feel better. But there is no such thing as a quick fix. There is one habit—leading an active lifestyle—that comes as close to that magic cure as we can get.

People who exercise regularly, when compared to those who don't exercise, decrease their chances of developing diabetes by 30 to 50 percent. Can you believe it? Just by getting active, you can cut your chances of developing diabetes in half. But how does exercise help? Exercise works by improving your body's ability to use insulin. People with type 2 diabetes tend to be insulin resistant, which means their bodies don't use insulin efficiently. Exercise can change all that.

Exercise can also reduce your body fat and prevent the loss of muscle mass that occurs every year as you age. How does this help? If you lose body fat, especially around your waistline, it can decrease your chances of developing diabetes. Also, the more muscle you have the more calories you burn because muscle burns more calories than fat. So you can eat more and still lose or maintain your weight, depending on what your goals are.

On top of all that, leading an active lifestyle helps you look and feel better. It causes cholesterol levels and blood pressure to drop. When you're consistently active, you sleep better, manage your stress better, have more energy to get things done, discover more self-confidence in what you do, and feel better about your body. So not only does activity add years to your life by reducing your chances of developing chronic diseases like diabetes, but it can add vitality to your years by improving your outlook on life.

So with all these benefits, why aren't we consistently more active as a society? One main reason is because we can't see and feel the benefits immediately. Other reasons are embarrassment, lack of coordination, dislike for our body shape, lack of time, or the initial discomfort of exercise. Yet, despite all these reasons, we know the payoff is there in the long run.

So to find you personal motivation, make a list of the benefits you'd like to receive from leading an active lifestyle and post it as a visual reminder of why you're trying to be active. As you experience the benefits, either add to the list or star those that remind you why you're doing what you're doing. Once you feel the benefits, you'll understand why this free miracle cure is so important.

~: 31 :~

A Few Minutes of Activity,
Here or There

Have you ever paid for a year's membership in a health club only to end up so overwhelmed with all the machines in the club or the intensity of the recommended workouts that you never enter the club after the first week? Often, we don't get moving because we think we have to do all high-intensity activities such as aerobics classes or running to reap any benefits. What we don't realize is that even a small amount of activity done consistently can add up to big health gains. For example, if the average person started walking one flight of stairs every day, after one year, he or she could lose six pounds. Small things, done *consistently*, really do add up.

Contrary to what many people think, you really don't need to join the high-intensity aerobics class to experience the health benefits of exercise. To improve your health and quality of life, you need a mere 30 minutes of activity per day. And you don't have to get all of the 30 minutes at once—it can be spread over the day.

What can count toward your 30 minutes of physical activity? Believe it or not, it can include simple things such as climbing the stairs, going for a brisk walk, raking leaves, cleaning the house, walking while talking on a portable phone, or getting up out of the lounge chair to change the television channel instead of using the remote control. Any daily activity counts. You just need to get at least 30 minutes over a day's time on all, or most, days of the week.

At this point, you might be saying, "I don't get it. What's the difference between physical activity and exercise?" Physical activity is any movement you do in the course of your daily living. Exercise, on the other hand, is a more vigorous type of activity that involves planned movements that are done specifically to improve your body composition (body fatness), flexibility, and muscular strength, as well as your heart and lungs. Jogging, step aerobics, weight lifting, stretching, calisthenics, swimming, and biking are just a few examples of exercise.

Physical activity and exercise both give you health benefits and improve your mood. If you're living an inactive lifestyle, you should start by focusing on physical activity—any activity that gets you moving. To see if you're getting 30 minutes or more on all, or most, days of the week, you may want to keep a log of your daily activities. If you're not at 30 minutes, find ways to get there. Some ideas are taking two trips to the washing machine, carrying in only one grocery bag at a time, or parking farther away in the parking lot at work. In the long run, these simple changes could be enough to prevent diabetes and to help you feel better about yourself while you're doing it.

◡ 32 ◡

Find Ways to Be Less Efficient

In today's fast-paced world, we work hard to be efficient at everything we do. We may take several loads of clothes to the laundry room at the same time, carry two bags of groceries at a time from the car, let the dog out in the backyard for activity instead of taking the dog for a walk. Is all this productivity good for our health?

Everyone wants to use time wisely, but what if being less productive was better for your health? Would you change your habits? Believe it or not, small changes in your daily routine can be the difference between meeting and not meeting your activity goals. So you may want to start looking for ways to get in some extra activity.

RETHINK THE EFFICIENCY HABIT

To be less efficient on a daily basis, consider trying the following:

- Walk around the block every time you get the mail.
- Pace when talking on a cordless telephone.
- Walk your dog instead of watching your dog walk.
- Take the stairs instead of the elevator.
- Hide the remote and walk to the television to change channels.

Weekly, some ways to get more activity could include the following:

- Stop at a park when out running errands to play with your children or to explore a trail.
- Be a little less efficient with housework—make extra trips when cleaning, doing laundry, or grocery shopping.
- Park at the far end of the parking lot when shopping.
- Mow the lawn then trim by hand instead of using an electric trimmer.
- Take extra trips when carrying out the trash.

Find ways to make monthly tasks less efficient:

- Wash your car by hand instead of taking it to an automatic car wash.
- Clean the attic, the basement, the closets.
- Trim trees and shrubs.
- Take an extra walk around the shopping mall before heading to the car.

These are only a few ideas to be less efficient on a daily, weekly, or monthly basis. With a little creativity, you can probably think of more. And the more you can think of and start doing, the more activity you're going to get on a daily basis. In the end, the less efficient you are in day-to-day activities, the more physical activity you'll get.

∿ 33 ∿

Pick Up the Pace with Exercise

Have you ever walked with someone who has a fast pace? Or have you tried to keep up with a certain pace on an exercise machine? Sometimes, keeping up with other people or machines feels uncomfortable at first because the pace isn't what we're used to.

Settling in to the routine of getting 30 minutes of physical activity is the first step, but there is a next progressive step to picking up the pace in your diabetes prevention plan—aerobic exercise. Just what is *aerobic* exercise? Any exercise that involves rhythmic motion of your arms and legs—biking, jogging, walking, cross-country skiing, in-line skating, swimming—and that is performed at a pace that temporarily increases your breathing and heart rate. It's recommended that you get aerobic exercise three to five times per week for 20 to 60 minutes.

Why include aerobic exercise? Because it improves your body's ability to use insulin, which may help prevent diabetes. Aerobic exercise also burns calories to help you manage your weight, strengthens your heart and lungs, and gives you endurance.

If you're not doing any aerobic exercise right now, it may be best to ease into it. In fact, if you haven't exercised in quite some time, check with your doctor before you begin. Then, start exercising by spreading your workouts throughout the week and doing only small amounts. For example, start out with 10 minutes, three times per week, and then increase the amount of time a few minutes each week until you get into the recommended range of 20 to 60 minutes. Once you're within that range, you can add another day or two to your routine.

How can you tell if you're exercising hard enough? Generally, you're breathing harder and you'll feel a little uncomfortable, in terms of going at a speed out of your normal pace. However, if you can't carry on a normal conversation while exercising, you're exercising too hard. Most likely, you've heard about measuring your heart rate to determine if your pace is fast enough. Another simpler way to measure if your pace is where it should be is to assess each workout on a scale of 1 to 20 with 1 being very, very light and 20 being very, very hard. Exercise should feel somewhat hard—but not strenuous—to maximize the benefits. On the 1 to 20 scale, this is around 13 to 15.

Before jumping right into an aerobic exercise workout, do a warm-up to get your body ready for exercise. A warm-up could include walking or biking slowly for a few minutes. After the warm-up, it's important to stretch your muscles for several minutes. This increases your flexibility and prepares your muscles for exercise, thus preventing injuries. After the aerobic exercise do a cool-down to slow your heart rate and to return your blood pressure to normal. Stretching again will reduce muscle soreness.

Keep in mind that when you start a new exercise routine, you work your muscles in a different way, which can lead to some stiffness or soreness for a day or two. This won't last for long after your body adjusts to the activities you choose. However, if you have any pain in muscles or joints that seems unusual or that persists for several days, contact your health care provider.

~: 34 :~

Strengthen Your Exercise Routine

We've probably heard or read that Americans don't exercise enough and that more and more of us are becoming overweight. But what we don't think about is that by not exercising, we lose about one-half to one pound of muscle each year. Why worry about losing muscle? Muscle is the calorie-burning engine of the body. So if we have less muscle, even if we eat the same amount of food, we can gain weight. Excess weight increases the odds that we'll get diabetes.

Strengthening exercises are often the missing link in an exercise routine. They can improve the body's use of insulin, prevent the loss of muscle, make bones stronger and rev up our metabolism. The more muscle we have, the more calories we'll burn. In fact, adding just one pound of muscle burns 30 to 50 extra calories per day. This could add up to 840 to 1,400 calories per month and 10,950 to 18,250 calories per year. Assuming we ate the same amount of food, this one pound of additional muscle means we'll lose three to five pounds per year. These are worthwhile numbers for those trying to lose weight to prevent diabetes.

What exercises give you this benefit? Strengthening exercises include calisthenics such as sit-ups and push-ups or weight training—working muscles against moderate resistance. The resistance can be provided by free weights (dumbbells or barbells or such household items as bottles of shampoo or cans of soup), resistance or rubber bands, or weight machines.

Before beginning these exercises, it's important to warm up for three to five minutes and then do stretching exercises. When you're finished exercising, cool down and stretch again. An exercise specialist at your health club or an exercise physiologist—

recommended by a health care provider—can help you set up a specific program to enhance your efforts even more. These professionals can teach you how to lift properly and can tell you the type and amount of weight to use. The ultimate goal is to do these exercises two to three times per week for about 15 to 20 minutes.

~: 35 :~

Juggle Your Exercise Program

Have you ever watched a juggler and wondered how he or she manages to toss numerous balls at once? Are there people you know who are great at juggling time? They have great time-management skills—somehow they manage to get everything done and still find time for themselves.

When you think about all the components of an exercise program—physical activity, aerobic exercise, and strengthening exercises—it can seem overwhelming. How can you fit it all into your schedule? Who has time to exercise every day? It may feel like you're being asked to climb Mount Everest at first. Yet once you get to the peak, it's all down hill from there.

The key is to start adding one activity at a time. Which activity comes first? It all depends on which one you're ready to begin doing. If you're more interested in aerobic exercise, start there. If it seems less threatening to work on the 30 minutes of daily activity, then that is the right starting point.

Once you've started doing one activity, it may be useful to think about how another could fit in. For example, when you do aerobic exercise, it's important to warm up your muscles and to stretch them before and after exercising to avoid an injury. Next, you could add strengthening exercises following an aerobic exercise session. This could include a few sit-ups, push-ups, or lifting weights or soup cans at the end of the session.

By adding strengthening exercises two or three times a week after aerobic exercise and getting a few minutes of daily activity here and there throughout your day, you balance your fitness routine. The key is to incorporate each activity into your schedule until you feel comfortable juggling all the balls.

～ 36 ～

Mind over Matter

Have you ever watched the movie *Field of Dreams*? It's about an Iowa farmer, Ray Kinsella, who hears the mysterious words "If you build it, he will come," and is compelled to build a baseball diamond in the middle of his cornfield. This farmer is thought by some to be a fool, or at least delusional. Yet his persistence is rewarded when spirits from baseball's past begin appearing on the ball field.

The story is about believing in ourselves, and it's also about persistence. And in that regard, although we may be motivated to start leading an active lifestyle, unless we do a little planning and develop a positive "I can do it" attitude, we may let the barriers we see stand in the way of the benefits we could realize.

You may be letting barriers stand between you and exercising. You can't wait for the barriers to magically disappear before you begin exercising—they never will disappear. You need to *plan* to overcome barriers to exercise. You need time, energy, and motivation to put exercise on your priority list and keep it there. Henry Ford had it right when he said, "Whether you think you can or you think you can't, you are right."

One way to ensure that you'll become more active is to think about the barriers that are keeping you from exercising. Here are some of the common barriers that many people face: What if I get injured? It takes too much energy to exercise. Wouldn't I have to spend a lot of money buying equipment or joining a health club? In today's fast-paced world, who has the time to exercise?

So how can you overcome any barriers that prevent you from exercising? First, you need to believe that you can exercise. You don't need to be Jane Fonda or Arnold Schwarzenegger to exercise. Second, you should focus on the benefits you will receive from exercise. Third, you can look for solutions to your barriers. It helps to make a mental or written list of all the reasons you're not exercising on a regular basis. For each barrier, think of some solutions. For example, if one of your barriers is that you feel too tired to exercise after work, think about when you could exercise. Could you exercise in the morning before work, or how about during your lunch hour? Could you stop at the park on the way home from work? Maybe your barrier is affordability. You don't need a health club membership to exercise. Go to a mall and walk. Buy an exercise video that you can do at home. Get a wind trainer for your bicycle and set it up indoors for the winter.

Whatever barriers you see, it's important to believe that you can overcome them. It truly is mind over matter. If you believe you can, then you can. If you believe it's impossible, it will be.

~: 37 :~

Map Out Your Exercise Program

When you take a road trip to a new and distant destination, do you just hop on the freeway without checking your map? Or do you research the most effective way to get to your end destination, plan out the mileage each day, and determine when and where you'll stop? Planning an activity-and-exercise schedule is similar to planning a road trip—you need to figure out your end destination and plan how you'll get there.

To map out your program, start by writing your ultimate goal at the bottom of a sheet of paper. Above that, in a line going across the paper, write some short-term goals that can help you get to your ultimate goal. Above each short-term goal, write a few weekly action steps that can help you achieve your short-term goals. This is where you will start. For example, will you walk three times a week for 20 minutes? Will you do 15 sit-ups two days per week? Think about how you'll incorporate these steps, as well as aerobic and strengthening exercises, into your day-to-day activities.

Next you may want to pull out your schedule and map out some time to accomplish these goals and action steps. When you plan a trip, it's easy to figure out the number of hours you'll drive and spend at each destination. In your daily living, however, you don't always map out the time you want to spend on activities that will make you feel better and that will help you lead a healthier life. By blocking out small segments of time in your calendar, you make your health a priority. These appointments with yourself are just as important as planning vacations or other daily activities.

To prevent boredom on the trip, don't forget to vary the routine to keep it interesting. When you were a kid, or maybe now when you're with your kids, do you play games in the car when you're on a road trip to keep the trip interesting? In the same way, you should try to vary your exercise routine. If you walk all the time for your aerobic exercise, you'll want to vary the route, sometimes walk with someone, or alternate days of walking with days of biking. Or try a dancing, kick-boxing, or spinning class at the health club. Variety is the spice of life, and it helps to keep us consistent with exercise.

Finally, you may want to keep track of your exercise progress. Why is it that we log mileage for our car and get excited about the number of miles to the gallon the car gets, but we don't keep track of our personal progress with our goals, and we don't celebrate milestones? Keep a journal of your exercise each week so you can see your progress in black and white. You can even mark your progress on a real map. Try picking a destination and track minutes as miles or track the actual miles walked. For fun, celebrate your success once the final destination is reached. Exercise can be like any road trip you take—it requires planning, flexibility, and some fun and games to keep you going.

SIMPLE CHANGES JOURNAL

What small changes can you make *today* to get more active?

What small changes can you make *this week* to get more active?

What small changes can you make *this month* to get more active?

✨ PART SIX ✨

Balance Your Lifestyle

In the year 2000, about 74 percent of households will be dual income. Amidst work, family responsibilities, and community involvement, we can get frustrated with the lack of time we can find to make our health a priority. But you can make it all fit in. You can find a way to strike a balance in your life in order to prevent diabetes.

~: 38 :~

Focus on the Whole You—
Body, Mind, and Spirit

Have you ever walked into a house—whether it's your own or that of a friend—and known immediately that you'd be comfortable there? The look, the layout, the smell, the history, the air—something about it all just felt right. The combined effect made you feel safe, warm, relaxed, at home.

And that is how you want to feel as you work toward building a healthier lifestyle—relaxed with a sense of balance and a feeling of comfort, and not stressed about possibly getting diabetes or finding time to fit exercise and healthful eating into your already busy days. And you can have this. But to do it, you need to think of yourself as you do the comfortable house. Having a healthier lifestyle isn't just about creating a better physical you with stronger muscles and fewer pounds, it's about the whole you—body, mind, and spirit. Just as the feeling you had in that house was a result of the whole package, managing health is a combined effort.

And when you think about it, focusing on the whole you makes sense. It is a fact that stress can contribute to heart disease and can cause migraine headaches, that depression can affect the immune system, and that your attitude about life can affect the number of aches and pains you feel. So as you find a balance in your life that includes taking care of your physical health, you must remember to be taking care of your mental well-being, too.

But how do you do this? How do you find the right balance in your life? Take a look at the sense of balance in your life as it is today by considering if you have the three things it takes to have balance: (1) a sense of contribution, (2) self-care, and

(3) a solid support system. Ask yourself the following questions to assess the balance in your life.

Sense of Contribution—Solid Ground:
- What are you passionate about?
- Do you have work that energizes you?
- Do you feel like you're making a significant contribution to your family, your company, or your community?
- Do you feel connected to the world around you?

Self-Care—Building the Foundation:
- Can you make a list of ten things that you personally enjoy doing?
- When was the last time you did something just for yourself?
- Do you know how much sleep your body needs to feel refreshed in the morning?
- Do you get the necessary amount of sleep most nights of the week?
- Are you physically active?
- Are you currently volunteering any of your time to a cause or an organization?
- When was the last time you talked to your neighbors?
- The bottom line is, are you taking care of you?

Solid Support System—Day-to-Day Maintenance:
- Are there people you can talk to about your experiences—both positive and negative?
- Do you have others who help you with household and family responsibilities?
- Do you know and routinely use any relaxation techniques such as deep breathing or yoga?

Thinking through these questions can help you assess whether you have a sense of balance in your life. If you're feeling out of balance, think about that house again. What would it take to find that place of comfort within you? To find success in managing your general health or, more specifically, in preventing diabetes or losing weight, it takes physical and mental well-being.

∿ 39 ∿

Monitor Your Stress

Stress is one of those words that always brings with it a nega-tive connotation. "My boss is stressing me out, and I'm not getting anything done at work." "I'm too stressed with every-thing else in my life to take time to exercise." "When I get tense, the first thing I do is reach for a tub of ice cream." Stress is prob-ably the one thing that makes us feel most like our lives are out of balance.

But keep in mind that the goal here is not to eliminate all stress from our lives. Some stress is good; it keeps us motivated, challenged, and satisfied. Life would be boring without it. As in many areas of health, however, moderation is the key. Too much stress is damaging to our health and can result in muscle tension, headaches, and stomach problems. Chronic stress can lead to serious health problems like heart disease and increased blood glucose levels. Not only is our physical well-being affected by stress, but also our mental health, relationships, and work performance.

The goal in achieving life balance, then, is to minimize and to manage the factors that add stress to your life. In general there are four main categories of stressors:

1. Environmental—pollution, traffic, noise, weather
2. Social—marriage or divorce, finances, job strain, death of a loved one
3. Physiological—sleep disorders, aging, menopause, living with a chronic disease
4. Internal—perfectionism, self-esteem issues, personality traits

The tricky thing about stress factors is that they are very individual. You may feel overwhelmed by last minute deadlines, whereas your co-worker thrives in that kind of environment. By the same token, an announcement that your parents are getting divorced might not affect you as much as it does one of your siblings.

So even though there are general categories of what causes anxiety for people, it's important to get more personal. If you've got a pretty good idea of what causes your stress level to rise, you can move on to the next step and figure out how you can manage these issues. If you're not sure about what stresses you out, you may want to create your own stress monitor log. For several days when you find yourself biting your finger nails or rubbing the tension out of your neck, jot down events that just happened. Consider things like a traffic jam on the way to work, financial problems (a worrisome bill just arrived in the mail), lack of sleep, unrealistic expectations of yourself, or marital problems.

Taking the time to identify the stressors in your own life can really be enlightening. You may not have previously realized the specific issues that were adding tension to your life, but now you will. Awareness of these stress factors gives you the information you need to move on to the next step—minimizing and managing stressors.

∻ 40 ∽

Lighten Your Stress Load

Identifying the stressors in your life is the first step toward minimizing them. But how do you minimize them? The following ideas have been useful for others trying to cope with tensions, to manage personal stressors, and to work toward a balance in life. You may want to try some of these *stress managers:*

- *Keep a time log.*   Poor time management can contribute to stress. To improve time-management skills, keep a log of how you're spending your time. Log your entries in quarter-hour, half-hour, or hour time blocks. Logging actions for a week or two can help you realize where time is wasted in your day and where you can simplify actions and steps. Furthermore, you'll have a better handle on how long tasks and projects actually take so you can plan more appropriately in the future.

- *Change how you react to situations.*   Although circumstances and people may not change, you always have the option of changing your reaction to them.

- *Get a massage.*   Whether from a professional massage therapist, family member, or friend, even a five-minute back or shoulder rub can relieve tension and stress, helping you to relax.

- *Exercise.*   Not only does exercise provide an immediate stress break, but it also lightens your mood by releasing endorphins into your bloodstream.

- *Learn to delegate.* While others might not do it exactly like you do, consider what tasks can be delegated to kids, partner, roommate, or co-workers.

- *Separate work and home.* You may leave one set of stressors at the office only to be met with varied family and household responsibilites when you walk in the door of your home. Between work and home, find 15 to 20 minutes to mentally and emotionally transition to the new environment.

- *Write "To Do" lists.* At the start of the day, make a list of everything that needs to be accomplished that day. Prioritize the tasks. Then cross off the lowest priority items on the list and move ahead with a realistic plan for the day.

- *Learn to say "no."* Before agreeing to take on a project, you should ask yourself how you feel about the request being made. Do you really want to do it? Do you know what you're being asked to do? Refuse without feeling guilty or making excuses if it's something you're really not interested in doing or if you can't commit yourself to the time and work involved.

- *Laugh.* A big belly laugh that brings you close to tears completely relaxes your body, distracts you from the stressor, and sheds new light on the situation.

- *Stretch during your work day.* Take a few minutes for shoulder rolls, toe touches, and side bends to relax your muscles and to give your mind a refreshing break.

- *Sleep.* Find the amount of sleep you need to be at your best, and get it every night.

✦ 41 ✦

Who Supports Your Efforts?

Remember learning how to ride a bike? If you were like most kids, you probably started with training wheels. The tiny wheels supported your bicycle while you learned the art of balancing while pedaling. Each day you rode, your balance got a little better. Soon you felt ready—or at least more confident in your ability—to ride without the extra support, and your parents took off the training wheels.

Trying to lead a healthier life to lower our chances of getting diabetes is similar to learning how to ride a bike. Initially we need to train ourselves to build lifestyle habits, and the training is easier if we have some support. Then, as we feel more confident about our new lifestyle, we need less assistance to maintain our new habits and keep the momentum going.

Just as training wheels balance your bike, a support system helps balance your life. You need to think about who your training wheels are. Who is there to support you as you work to build healthier habits?

To answer this question, take a blank sheet of paper and on it draw a bike wheel that has 12 to 16 spokes. In the center of the wheel (the hub), write your name. Then begin filling the spokes of the wheel with names of the people to whom you look for support—a spouse or a partner, siblings, parents, other relatives, friends, co-workers, health care providers, health club staff. Who are the people to whom you go to discuss health-related problems? Does someone help out around the house and with the kids? Are there people you know who are also interested in health? On whose shoulder do you cry? Who would you call to have a celebration?

How many spokes did you fill? If not many, your circle of

support may have weak spots, and you may need to build on this as you work to become successful at managing weight and preventing diabetes. If you have several spokes filled in, your balance and confidence and likelihood for success in managing your health are high.

Working toward a healthier lifestyle isn't always easy. You need to feel comfortable with the level of support—your training wheels—that you'll have as you develop positive health behaviors.

~: 42 :~

Find the Support You Need

Many of us are used to being independent, resourceful people. And we may be the one providing support for our children, our aging parents, and our friends. If that is so, it may be difficult for us to be the ones asking for support, telling others what we need from them and how they can help us.

Yet this is exactly what we need to do. To be successful at changing health habits, we need to build a strong support system. There are two steps to gaining the support we need: (1) find supportive partners and (2) teach others how they can support us.

As you work to change lifestyle habits, you'll derive many benefits from having supportive people in your life. They can encourage you, empathize with you, and just listen to the struggles you're having as you change eating or exercise habits. A partner can motivate you and keep up your momentum by offering to exercise with you. Supportive people can help you day in and day out, not just when things have gotten you down.

A support person—whether it's a spouse, a significant other, or a friend—should be a person with whom you feel comfortable sharing your concerns and goals about diabetes prevention. It's helpful to think about these attributes when choosing a truly supportive partner:

97

Aттributes for a Support Person

- Easy to talk to about health goals or setbacks
- Expresses concern about his or her own health
- Understands the difficulties of managing weight and health
- Displays a genuine interest in helping you
- Thinks positively—the glass is half full not half empty
- Provides encouragement on a regular basis

If you have someone in your life who has most or all of these attributes, you've probably found an ideal support person. If you can't think of anyone who fits the description, seek out someone who has these characteristics. Keep in mind that no one person can provide all the support you need. It takes many people to build a strong circle of support—to keep your training wheels properly attached and inflated.

If you're interested in enhancing your circle of support, seek out people who have similar goals or issues. Being around others who are going through the same thing as you are is a validating experience. It's nice to know you're not alone. If you like groups, there are options like Weight Watchers or TOPS (Take Off Pounds Sensibly) for weight management. You can join a local health club, a mall-walking program, or a community education class. The options are endless; what you choose depends on what your needs are.

◡ 43 ◡

Help Your Support System Help You

Just because you interact with many people on a daily basis—spouse, kids, co-workers—doesn't always mean that those people will know what you need from them. So as you build your support system, there are times when you'll need to teach others how to support you. Different people will have different reactions to changes you're making for your health. Your kids, for example, might resent the new low fat dinners you're serving. Friends who also have health issues may feel threatened by the positive changes you make. If you suddenly start saying no to outside commitments so you can make health a priority, many people may struggle with the shift in you.

So it's important to work with others to help them understand how they can support you as you change your lifestyle. Consider the following ways to become more effective at getting support from others:

- *Express yourself.* Don't be afraid to tell others what's on your mind. Get specific about how they can help you and motivate you. Use words that describe your feelings instead of neutral terms when sharing your thoughts. When communicating with your supportive partners, use the words "I think" or "I feel."

- *Learn to feel comfortable talking about yourself.* You probably tend to downplay your accomplishments and successes, but it's okay to share your health achievements with family and friends. It's also important to be open about your frustrations and struggles.

- *Make eye contact.* Even if you're discussing an uncomfortable topic, try to look people directly in the eye when talking to them.

- *State disagreements.* Just because they're supporting you in this new endeavor doesn't mean that you always have to agree with your partner. When letting your partner know about an area of disagreement, again use statements like "I think," "I feel," or "I have a different outlook on that matter."

- *Acknowledge others when they give you support.* When you tell them how much you appreciate them and their help, they'll be more likely to continue with their support. It's a win-win situation for both of you—you get support and they get the satisfaction of helping someone and being appreciated for their help.

∽ 44 ∾

Talk Yourself into Healthier Habits

Have you ever thought about why advertising campaigns are so effective? "Just do it." "Baseball, hot dogs, apple pie, and Chevrolet." "It's the real thing." Each slogan evokes an emotional response to the product. We can quickly name each product, because Nike, Chevrolet, and Coca-Cola have repeated their slogans to us frequently in attempts to sway our emotions so we'll purchase their products.

The same is true of our own thoughts and ideas. We're constantly generating thoughts about ourselves—our health, our body size and shape, and our competency in work and relationships. Because we hear these same thoughts or messages all the time, they establish our attitudes and feelings about ourselves. In the end, this self-image that is created affects our actions and whether we succeed or fail in various areas of our lives. For example, every time you look in the mirror, you may say to yourself, "No matter how much weight I lose, I'll never get rid of this gut!" Repeated in your mind enough times, this thought lowers your self-image and confidence, affecting your motivation to lose weight.

The previous self-message was negative, but you can also send yourself positive messages. Unfortunately, since childhood, most of us have learned from society to downplay our own abilities, skills, and talents. Because of this, you may doubt your capablities and underestimate your self-worth as an adult. All these negative thoughts take root in your subconscious, making you uncertain about how you can keep off the lost weight or making you question whether you can maintain the day-to-day routine necessary to improve your health.

But you can reverse this uncertainty by reprogramming your subconscious with a technique called self-talk. It's as simple as the name implies. By verbalizing positive messages frequently and continually, you can retrain your mind to be motivated, energized, and on track with diabetes prevention and weight management (or any other area of your life where you'd like to make some changes). You can overpower all those negative messages currently floating around in your mind.

If you're interested in improving your self-talk, listen to the messages you currently send yourself. Every time you make a negative statement or have a negative thought about yourself, write it down in a notebook, your daytimer, or a wipe board posted on the refrigerator. Do this for one to two weeks. Negative self-talk can be subtle, so listen closely to the messages. Some examples of negative messages are:

"I can't do it."

"Why should I try? It probably won't work anyway."

"I've never been successful at losing weight before. Why should this time be any different?"

"I know he/she won't like me."

"I'm just not good at athletics."

Once you have a list of negative self-talk messages, categorize them. Do most relate to your body size and shape? To your health? To your job performance? Categorizing the messages will give you an idea of where to start. Suppose you choose to work on negative health-and-body messages, even though they're not the most frequent. (It's best to work on just one area of self-talk at a time.)

Next, review the chosen category of negative messages. It can then be helpful to write some positive statements to counter them. (Another easy way to do this is to write negative messages on one side of recipe cards and the corresponding positive messages on the other.) Make your positive statements simple and

clear and consistent with the health goals you've set. Examples
of positive self-talk to combat some of the negative messages
mentioned earlier are:

Negative	Positive
Why should I try? It probably won't work anyway.	I'll try, and I acknowledge that I may have to try several times before I succeed.
I've never been successful at losing weight before. Why should this time be any different?	Today is the first day of the rest of my life. I can take charge of my weight by taking one day at a time.
I know he/she won't like me.	I have many likeable characteristics and traits. People will enjoy meeting and getting to know me.

Once you've written your positive messages, it's best to keep
them with you throughout the day as a constant reminder.
Writing them on note cards, posting them on your bathroom
mirror or computer screen, or recording them on a cassette tape
that can be played back several times during the day makes the
new messages really come alive.

When you first start practicing the art of self-talk, there will
be some internal arguments between your old and your new
programming. To win the argument, positive messages need to
be repeated frequently. Saying them out loud is most effective
because another sense—your hearing—becomes involved in
the process. It may take several weeks for the positive self-talk
to take over, but it will be worth the effort to give you new confidence to achieve your goals.

∿ 45 ∿

Visualize Success

Have you ever seen the movie *Brian's Song*? It's about a professional football player named Brian Piccolo who gets cancer. But he fights back against the pain by using his mind— letting it take control over his physical body. This technique is called *creative visualization,* and it involves using images to combat negative thoughts. Actors use imagery to really get inside a role. Professional athletes use it to get energized and to push themselves to work harder. More and more it's being prescribed as part of pain management for people with chronic disease. And it may be your answer to finding a balance between physical health and mental well-being.

If you're interested in trying creative visualization, begin by finding a quiet spot to relax. Using one of your negative self-messages (for example, I have to work out five days a week for exercise to really make any difference, and I don't have that kind of time), follow these three steps:

1. *Set an action step.* One example is: I will start getting active by working out two days a week after I get home from work.

2. *Create an image in your mind of how you'd like the situation to be.* For example, if you find you're procrastinating about working out, create an image in your mind of how you would make it happen. Imagine yourself driving home from work and anticipating how good it will feel to get your body moving. Have you already decided what activity you'll do? How long will your workout be? Once you arrive home,

what do you do? Do you immediately get changed into workout clothes? Imagine yourself starting the activity. Can you see the stress just leaving your body as you continue the workout? Can you see how much stronger you're becoming? Don't your legs feel great? After the workout, picture yourself feeling refreshed and energized. Let the sweat trickle down you as a reminder of the calories you've burned. Feel the muscles in your body pulsing with strength and renewed vigor. As you create the image in your mind, remember to keep your image in the present, not the future.

3. *Focus on this image often.* Once you have the image detailed, commit it to memory. Then every chance you get, think of it. In quiet moments before you fall asleep at night, during your morning shower, and as frequently as you can throughout the day, replay this image.

Be patient with creative visualization. It may take some time for the new image to take root, but you'll begin to notice a change in your attitude about how you manage your health. This technique is proof positive that total health is a mind-body connection.

Simple Changes Journal

What small changes can you make *today* to find a sense of balance in your life?

What small changes can you make *this week* to find a sense of balance in your life?

What small changes can you make *this month* to find a sense of balance in your life?

✣ PART SEVEN ✣

Make Diabetes Prevention a Family Affair

You know that one of the main factors leading to diabetes is heredity. Your chances of getting diabetes are related to its incidence in your family. Usually you have more in common with your family than just heredity, too. You often share the same lifestyle habits and routines. So there's a great advantage to getting the entire family involved in making positive lifestyle changes. Diabetes prevention—it's a family affair.

∿ 46 ∿

Turn Your Family On to Health

Have you ever read stories in popular magazines about families who have lost 500 pounds among them all? Or sisters who started rowing together to get in shape? Or father-son teams who ran their first marathon together? Well, the next story could be yours to tell. You could have the family that turns their health around to prevent diabetes and other chronic diseases. All it takes is making health a family affair.

There are many reasons to get the other people who live in your household—or maybe even family members not in your household—as motivated as you are about changing their lifestyle. First, because you are all related, your relatives may have many of the same risk factors for diabetes that you do. So you'll all benefit from getting active, managing weight, or eating better. Even if you're not blood relations, you probably have many lifestyle habits that are the same if you live in close proximity to each other. Building healthier habits with these people makes it easier for all of you to stay on track.

Having a partner or multiple partners with similar goals can provide a tremendous amount of support for your efforts to build healthier habits. You won't have to try to roll out of bed in the morning when it's still dark outside. Now there will be someone to drag you out and to take that walk before work with you. Beer-and-pizza night can still be a dinner out, but it can revolve around a more nutritious choice, like a smaller size pizza with a thick crust and vegetable toppings. And now, you'll have someone to celebrate your successes with.

There's also an advantage to getting the young members of your household involved in better health, too. Kids can make anything fun—bike riding, in-line skating, and skipping rope.

If they're raised on healthful eating habits, they're likely to continue with these habits into adulthood. Getting them hooked on lifetime sports like tennis, golf, and bowling that can be done as a fun family activity is a great starting point. You'll be helping them as well as yourself to build healthy behaviors that you can continue indefinitely.

If you're thinking about getting your family involved in health, you might find that you're the one who has thought the most about preventing diabetes. If this is true, it may be up to you to take a lead role in getting others involved—whether they're in your immediate family or in your extended family. You can do this by encouraging anyone who is interested to assess his or her chance of getting diabetes. Try talking about risk factors that you have in common or about ideas for things you can do together to lower the risk of diabetes for everyone who's involved. Another idea is to brainstorm healthful changes in your family events—pot lucks and picnics where the goal is to bring all low fat items, cross-country ski excursions after you eat that Thanksgiving turkey, or family vacations biking through Yellowstone Park.

The bottom line is that family members, whether they live with you on a daily basis or have been one of your supports since childhood, can reap many benefits by making diabetes prevention a family affair.

❧ 47 ❧

Plant Your Family Health Tree

Many people are interested in geneology—the study of their family tree. After all, looking into their ancestors can tell them a great deal about their families as they exist today. How did Aunt Gertrude get her name? Who did that one niece inherit her red hair from? Why did Grandma and Grandpa settle in Maine rather than anywhere else in the country?

But what if we take our family trees one step further by creating a health tree? It is believed that there are over 5,000 inheritable diseases, and diabetes is definitely one of them. A family health tree is one way to determine if, and how far back, diabetes extends into our families. This information can give us a much clearer picture of our chance of getting diabetes as well as that of our children and grandchildren.

To develop your own family health tree, all you need are the tactics used by any good reporter: who, what, when, where, and how.

- *Who.* Because your chances of having diabetes and weight problems are affected by your genetics, tracking health information on blood relatives (parents, grandparents, aunts, uncles, sisters, brothers) as far back as you can tells you more about your risk. Even though spouses of blood relations tell less of the story, it's still a piece of the puzzle. For example, if an uncle by marriage died of diabetes complications, it can provide insight to the lifestyle habits he and your aunt shared (were they inactive, for example, which contributed to him getting diabetes?).

- *What.* Gather information on your ancestors' causes of death, illnesses prior to death, chronic diseases, problems during pregnancy (gestational diabetes, birth of a large baby), physical description (height, weight, ethnic background), lifestyle habits (life work that was or wasn't physically demanding, eating habits), and medications they used. These pieces of information paint a picture of why someone did or didn't get diabetes. You may need to ask probing questions to get a real picture of some lifestyle habits. After all, our mothers didn't go to the gym to get their exercise. They scrubbed floors by hand, gardened, walked to the grocery store, and hung clothes out on the line for activity. Without asking these questions, you may not realize that this high level of activity may have prevented them from developing diabetes.

- *When.* How old were your family members when they died? When did they first get a chronic disease or illness? What were the dates of their deaths? How do these dates coincide with medical advances for particular diseases, especially diabetes?

- *Where.* To fill out the branches and leaves on your family health tree, consider where ancestors lived out their lives. Was it in another country? If so, were there wars and natural disasters that increased their chances of developing certain diseases? Historically, certain diseases have started in one culture and been passed to others through marriages or adoption of lifestyle habits of that culture. For example, many people eat more fat when they move to a Western country like the United States. More fat can translate to extra weight and a higher chance of getting diabetes. Knowing whether they lived in a rural or an urban area is also useful information because it can indicate their access to health care.

- *How.* To gather this information on your family, review death certificates and medical records. Family stories passed down over the years or interviews with older relatives can fill in the gaps. An invaluable resource is a medical dictionary. It can be useful when trying to understand the varying terms that may all point to the same disease. For example, carcinoma, malignancy, and osteosarcoma all mean cancer.

Although you may not be able to gather as much information as you'd like on all your ancestors, fill in as many of the details as possible. The more you have, the clearer will be the picture of the strength of your own root system. With what you learn through your family health tree, you can prevent history from repeating itself by making lifestyle changes where they're most necessary.

~: 48 :~

Use Body Silhouettes to Track History in the Making

What would happen to your family tree if you changed everything that's within your power to change? Would there be more branches? A stronger root system? More rings in the stump indicating an increased tree age? Although you can't change what happened in the past, you can impact what is happening today and in the future.

You've already looked into the health of your ancestors, but now it's time to look at the health history you're creating on a daily basis—and not just for yourself, but for your entire family. This information will be useful for generations to come, but it's also helpful to look at what you have in common with others living in your household. It may show how you can support one another to change history in the making.

If you're interested in doing so, body silhouettes are a great way to track your health on an ongoing basis. To use this tool, draw a simple but realistic outline of your body on a fairly large, blank sheet of paper. To reflect your current weight and apple versus pear body shape, it's important that the outline be realistic. Shade in body parts that have been injured during your lifetime (e.g., an arm that was broken), and organs that may be adversely affected (e.g., your heart if you have high blood cholesterol). Jot down brief notes with the date the health problem occurred or was diagnosed. Try to include some notes as well on lifestyle habits, for example, whether you exercise routinely or if you smoked for 10 years and have since quit.

Don't forget to get everyone in your household involved in body silhouettes, including your kids. Although they may seem too young to start worrying about their risk of chronic diseases like diabetes, the more complete their silhouette, the more health clues it will provide in the future. And besides, they'll have fun with it, too.

As you work on your body silhouette over the years, periodically compare it to your family health tree. Are there similarities you can find with your ancestors? Does your body size and shape seem similar to a grandparent who died of diabetes complications? This tool is just one more way you can prevent history from repeating itself.

∿ 49 ∿

Individuals Make Up the Family Team

Are you a type-A personality? Are you a Virgo or a Pisces? Does "extrovert" or "introvert" describe you better?

There are many different ways to type personalities, work styles, and decision-making styles. So when you embark on health as a family affair, it's important to take each personality and style into consideration. Who in the group is the cheerleader? Who is the organizer? Is one person more likely to procrastinate? Are you a morning person married to a night owl? Knowing these things about your family health team allows you to use them to your advantage and increases the likelihood that you'll find success in building healthy habits and preventing diabetes.

Bear in mind, too, that some family members will be more ready to change various lifestyle behaviors than others will. But this can have a truly positive effect on the success of the family working together. If, for example, you're planning to add aerobic exercise to your weekly routine, a sister, a teenage daughter, or a spouse who is already exercising may be just the partner for you. In another area of health, such as stress management, you might be the one doing the encouraging and the motivating.

You've probably encountered many different ways of typing individuals in various areas of your life, and there are also different defined personalities when it comes to working together as a family on health. Considering each of the following types may give you a better view of who is in on your family affair of health.

Fatalists believe they're victims. Whatever health problems were dealt to them, they are stuck with them, and there's nothing they can do about it. These people may smoke or not worry about other less-than-healthful behaviors because they don't believe their actions can really affect their future. "If I'm going to get diabetes, I'm going to get diabetes" is their attitude.

Skeptics also believe that the cards have already been dealt, but their response to this is much different. They're willing to work hard at getting and staying healthy. They exercise, make nutritious food choices, and have a sense of balance in their lives, but at the same time believe their efforts are in vain. They also feel that any present knowledge about prevention may be found to be totally wrong in the future.

Fighters refuse to accept the hand they were dealt and believe they can overcome risk of disease. Hard work, they believe, will absolutely pay off in the end. They're dedicated to prevention and are often willing to try alternative as well as traditional therapies to improve health.

In any family, you're likely to find a mix of these health personalities. But again, the mix can be used to the family's advantage. Maybe the fatalist in your group is the right person to gather statistics and other information that will be useful. The skeptic may be assigned to make a list of the benefits of making lifestyle behavior changes. Keeping the group motivated is up to the fighters.

Whether we're looking at these health personalities, at stages of change, or at other personality profiles, success as a group is definitely dependent on using the strengths that we all bring to the party to outweigh the weaknesses and realities that we all have.

⌁ 50 ⌁

Kids: They're Never
Too Young to Get Involved

Ah, youth. Do you remember yours? The fun you had. The games you played. The experimentation you did. The crowds you ran with. Youth is definitely a time to have fun—to just play. Do you see this in your own children, nieces, nephews, grandchildren, or other kids you know? Although the games may have changed, kids still love to have fun. Think of the laughter that rings throughout the house, the energy kids have, the long attention span when it comes to doing something they enjoy.

Because most of us have fond memories of our youth, we hate to do anything to break the spell for any child. But children can get started on healthful habits and still have fun. We don't need to mention the words *diabetes* or *disease* or the fact that many diseases start years before they're ever diagnosed. We know all of this, but our kids don't have to. All they need is help building healthy habits that will last a lifetime.

One area toward which you can guide your kids for a lifetime of health and disease prevention is activity. The range of sports in which kids can participate is wider than ever, and it is important to give some thought to the choices made. Football, basketball, and soccer are always popular, but are they sports that your kids can play for the rest of their lives? Typically, young people can find organized leagues for these sports through high school or maybe college, but after that they might have a difficult time finding a league in which to play their sport. Then they're left not knowing what to do for activity. On the other hand, tennis, golf, and biking are activities for people of any age and in almost any place. If people start these activities when they are young, they'll build skill in these activities and, most likely, continue with them into adulthood.

Healthful eating habits is the other area in which you want to start your children young. Children *over age two* can be started on low fat eating habits, and that is definitely the time to do it. Encourage them to eat plenty of fruits and vegetables, to eat when they're hungry and to stop when they're full, and to make low fat choices whenever possible. When taught young, these eating habits will be their normal pattern for the rest of their lives.

As you work to get your kids on a health kick, you should remember that role modeling has a huge impact on what kids learn. You can't have soft drinks with meals and expect your kids to drink milk. You can't sit watching television in the evening and expect your kids to go ride their bikes. Kids watch what adults do and mimic that behavior. It's up to you to make sure they have healthy habits to copy, like staying active and eating right.

Remember, health is a family affair. If you teach your children well—you will be giving them a long life without diabetes and other diseases.

~: 51 :~

Write a Health Contract

If you hire someone to build you a new house, you sign a contract. When you buy a brand new car, you check to make sure you have enough insurance coverage. If you work as a consultant, you're sure to have a signed agreement between yourself and the person or the company with whom you're consulting. So why would something as serious as your health and the health of your family be without a contract?

It shouldn't. Changes you make now can have a dramatic effect on how long you live and on the quality of your life. So to prove that your entire family is serious about making changes and sticking with them, it's best to spell it all out in black and white. It can be called a family contract, a health agreement, or whatever other name comes to mind. The important things to discuss are goals, plans, hopes, and fears about building a healthier lifestyle to prevent diabetes.

What can be included in a family health contract? Perhaps one of the most important things to include is the family's overall goal. Doing this means that in the future, decisions will be based on this goal. For example, a health-oriented family vacation may be chosen over a really decadent trip (like a cruise where food is constantly available); a push mower will be purchased instead of a riding lawn mower because using a push mower is better exercise; or a family membership to the YMCA will be fit into the monthly budget. If there are family members who have very specific goals, include those as well. Then other group members know the kind of support this individual will need.

If you decide that writing a family health contract will work for your family, consider setting up a review of the contract each year or every other year. This will force you to assess how you're doing, and it will also provide an opportunity to celebrate the success the family has had. And while you're at it, be sure to build in rewards. Hard work, commitment, and achievement of a goal deserve to be rewarded. As you complete your family contract, be sure to have everyone sign it, truly treating it as a binding agreement.

Simple Changes Journal

What can you do *today* to get your family involved in diabetes prevention?

What can you do *this week* to get your family involved in diabetes prevention?

What can you do *this month* to get your family involved in diabetes prevention?

PART EIGHT

Staying on Track with Your Diabetes Prevention Plan

Have you ever noticed all the positive reinforcement you get when you start building a healthier lifestyle? People notice the weight you've lost, the healthful lunches you've been making, or the fact that you're exercising more. All the attention and the action steps you've taken can be motivating. But how do you transition to maintaining your new health behaviors and stay motivated for the long haul? Working to prevent diabetes is a day-in, day-out, long-term project. Being flexible and committed can help you stay on track with diabetes prevention for a lifetime of good health.

~: 52 :~

Adapt to Change

We've all experienced change in our lives. Big changes like getting married, having a child, or adopting a pet are more notable because they instantly make our lives different. At first, these changes may seem overwhelming. But after a while, we adapt to them. In fact, once we adjust to changes, we often can't imagine how life would be without the changes—if we weren't married, or didn't have a child, or had never gotten a pet.

The same is true for changes in your eating or exercise habits. Once you modify your lifestyle, building permanent habits, it's hard to imagine life as it was before. Old behaviors start to feel uncomfortable. Skipping exercise or eating lots of high fat foods, for example, may feel awkward. These habits just don't fit or describe who you are anymore.

When you've reached the point where old habits don't feel comfortable, you're probably ready to transition from actively changing habits to maintaining new ones. This can also be an odd feeling, at least initially. Why? Because after spending months creating action steps to change how you eat, how much you exercise, or how much you weigh, it may feel like you're not accomplishing as much when you're just working to maintain the changes.

Yet in reality, maintenance is a positive aspect. It means you've accomplished numerous action steps, many short-term goals, and eventually, most of your long-term goals. You're one step closer to achieving your diabetes prevention plan.

❧ 53 ❧

Develop a Maintenance Contract

We take our cars to the shop for oil changes and tune-ups at certain mileage points. Each year we head to the doctor and the dentist for annual checkups. We develop our own schedules for maintaining our homes. It seems we have maintenance required for most of the major purchases in our lives.

Have you ever thought about creating a maintenance contract for diabetes prevention? A personal plan for better health could increase your chances of successfully maintaining the behaviors you've worked so hard to change.

Take New Year's resolutions, for example. Each year at least half of us make one or more. But most of us won't be successful at maintaining them. It's all in the numbers. At one week, 77 percent of us will be successful with our resolutions. At one month, 55 percent are successful. At six months, only 40 percent are successful, and after two years, only 19 percent. Would more of us have been successful if we had created a maintenance contract? Probably.

What could this contract include? When you purchase any major appliance or a vehicle, you usually get a warranty. This is the manufacturer's commitment to the product. One of the first things you can do is to keep your commitment to health. You want to commit to continuing to make the habits—the ones that can prevent diabetes—a priority. So the contract could include a few statements on why preventing diabetes is important to you.

Determining time frames to celebrate milestones is also an important component of your maintenance contract. Have you ever celebrated a child's clean bill of health at a checkup or a car that is working great despite the fact that it has 200,000 miles on it? Why not celebrate your present health and the goals you've achieved to improve your health? Reviewing your accomplishments helps you continue to renew your commitment to prevent diabetes.

Your maintenance contract could also include a support person. Maintaining lifestyle habits does require some help from others. You need someone to be there to celebrate successes or to pick you up when you have fallen down. Your support person could be the person with whom you develop a contract to review your diabetes prevention plan, to be on call for those times when you need to bend an ear, or to exercise or to eat nutritiously with you. The key is figuring out what kind of support you need and asking for it.

To maintain the momentum, you may want to think about creating a formal, written contract with yourself. Your health is much more valuable than your house or your car, so why not commit to making it a priority? Make your own personal warranty for diabetes prevention.

❧ 54 ❧

Know Your Limits

"Speed Limit—65 miles per hour."
"You can have two cookies after dinner."
"Bedtime is 9 P.M."
"I have only 15 minutes to discuss that."
"I can have two drinks at dinner."
"I won't spend more than $75 for boots."
Maximum dosage: 12 teaspoons (of cough medicine) in 24 hours.

Every day, you encounter situations of limits with yourself and with your family, friends, and co-workers. Some limits you impose, some are imposed on you.

We usually view any type of limit negatively. We all want to do what we want and when we want, right? But if there weren't any limits, what type of structure would there be in our lives? Would the streets be safe to drive on without speed limits? Don't children do better with a consistent routine? Limits don't have to have a negative concept. They just help define some boundaries. Think about signs for speed limits. The signs typically list a minimum and a maximum speed limit.

Eating healthier and exercising to prevent diabetes and manage weight are no different—they require setting some limits. You may try to monitor portions, limit high fat foods, or watch less television so you become more active. But once you've developed positive lifestyle habits, the limits don't stop. New types of limits begin.

As you move forward, continuing to change lifestyle habits and to maintain the ones you've already developed, it's important that you set limits for yourself. For example, if you lost weight and started gaining weight again, at what point would you act? Three pounds? Five pounds? If you missed several days of walking or stopped eating fruits and vegetables, when would you get back on track? Would you let your habits go for one week? Would you start again in one month?

When you set limits for yourself in advance, you have a plan. You know your boundaries, minimum and/or maximum. In a sense, it's like setting goals—you have a specific, measurable statement that tells you what actions you plan to take in a certain situation. The limits could relate to weight gain, eating, activity, or stress management.

As you consider limits, you also need to think about what action steps you'll take if you *exceed* your limits. An example of a limit and an action step is: "I will weigh myself once a week. If my weight increases by three to five pounds, I will monitor my food portions again." Another one is: "If I go more than one week without exercising, I will call a friend and set up a few appointments to exercise together."

Are there limits you'd like to set for yourself? You may want to take some time to think about them and make a mental or written note of them. By developing a plan in advance and outlining steps to take when lifestyle habits get off track, you're more prepared to continue your healthy habits for a lifetime.

∽ 55 ∾

Plan . . . Do . . . Check . . . Act

We make grocery lists so that our shopping trips to the grocery store are efficient—so we won't forget anything. Each day many of us create "To Do" lists so we can visualize all the things we want to get done that day or in the days to come. These types of lists help us feel organized. We know what we want to achieve.

In the working world, lists are taken a few steps further to keep things organized. For example, many companies now use a process called *continuous quality improvement* to improve work flow, services, or programs. This process involves planning, which is similar to list making, and doing, which is carrying out the plan. But it also involves checking the process to see if it worked and then acting to improve the quality or the efficiency of the process.

Maintaining lifestyle habits to prevent diabetes is similar to continuous quality improvement. In a sense, you've already been planning and doing. You might have planned to eat more fruits, and you're doing it. Maybe you wanted to exercise more, and now you are. If your goal was to lose a few pounds, you may have already lost the weight. It's great when you plan to make a change in your habits and then do it.

Yet as you begin to maintain your habits, you should have a plan in place for those times when you start to slip back into old habits. Or better yet, have a proactive plan to periodically check how you're doing and, if necessary, to continue to make changes in your lifestyle habits. One great way to do this is self-monitoring. By periodically recording your weight, exercise, and/or eating habits, you can assess whether there have been any new changes (positive or negative) in how you eat, how much you exercise, or in how much you weigh. The information not only helps you to see that there are changes but, after assessing it, can also help you determine what steps you'll take to get back on track or to stay on track.

To self-monitor, you can record your weight, stress level, and eating and/or activity habits in a notebook, in a journal, or on a computer. Some daily planners also have food or activity logs you can buy to use with them. Recording only those things that are meaningful to you is necessary. Maybe you want to know how well you're doing with your fat grams, so you record food items eaten, portion sizes, and fat grams. Are you getting the 30 minutes of physical activity each day? To determine if you are, try recording daily activities you do, and add up the minutes. Think about those areas on which you've been working in your diabetes prevention plan and assess how you're doing.

How often should you log your habits? You can do it every day, a few days a month, quarterly, or only when you feel you're starting to slip back into old behaviors. The nice part about self-monitoring is that you can do whatever fits your needs. The key is to continue checking how you're doing and acting when you feel it's necessary.

✌ 56 ✌

Keep the End in Mind

When you start a project, whether it's a report for work, a household task like painting, or a hobby like woodwork or needlepoint, do you only think about starting the project? Or do you visualize what the project will look like when completed?

Most often, we think about how we want the project to turn out, and we work backward—keeping the end in mind. The same is true for a diabetes prevention plan. Everything you do to lead a healthier life adds to your success. However, the key is staying motivated. Changing habits to prevent diabetes is a life-long effort. It's not a short-term project.

So how can you stay focused for the long haul? You can start by learning how others have made diabetes prevention their long-term project. Take Patsy from Connecticut, for example. She has two brothers and two sisters who died from the complications of diabetes. Her father and one of her mother's sisters had diabetes. So when her doctor told her that her blood glucose levels were high (impaired fasting glucose), she wasn't surprised. She was expecting it because of her strong family history.

What did she do? Her doctor told her that in order to prevent diabetes, she needed to eat healthier and to exercise. Since that time, she tries to exercise regularly and to make more nutritious food choices. Now her high blood glucose levels have returned to the normal range. And Patsy plans to keep it that way. She wants to live a long life and to avoid the complications of diabetes that her other family members experienced.

The lesson to learn from Patsy is that even though a strong family history of diabetes does increase your chances of getting the disease, you can influence the outcome. You don't always have to let nature take its course.

Jane from Boston is also working to prevent diabetes. When she was pregnant, her doctor told her she had gestational diabetes. She, like most women, had her blood glucose levels return to normal after the pregnancy. Yet she still has at least a one-in-four (or higher) chance of getting diabetes later in life.

How does Jane stay motivated to prevent diabetes? She focuses on all the benefits she feels on a day-to-day basis. When she's consistent with her exercise, she feels less stressed. Going for walks and being active with her two sons give her two benefits in one—health benefits and quality time with her kids. So by reviewing all the short-term benefits, you can stay focused, eventually achieving your long-term project—diabetes prevention.

The bottom line is that you have to keep the end in mind—preventing diabetes—so you don't lose focus during this very long-term project. Remembering why you're doing what you're doing and focusing on the benefits of your actions can keep you motivated for a long, healthy life.

⌁ 57 ⌁

Even the Best-Laid Plan Isn't Foolproof

Whether it's planning a wedding, a project at work, or our retirement, we try to think through all the possible "what if" scenarios so we can be prepared for the unexpected. This makes our plan complete and ensures that in the long run we're successful at reaching our goal.

But even the best-laid plan can go awry. It's impossible to predict everything that could potentially happen. Sometimes factors beyond our control interfere with our plan and prevent us from reaching our goal.

The same applies to your diabetes prevention plan. Even the best-laid plan isn't foolproof. Although you've worked at building positive habits like exercising, managing stress and your weight, and making nutritious food choices, you may need to do more. Genetics or other factors may take over, causing you to develop diabetes despite your efforts. However, by having a plan and working to prevent diabetes, you most likely delayed getting it by at least a few years and improved your quality of life—both now and later. Early identification of diabetes and leading a healthier life helps you avoid the more serious complications of the disease that happen when diabetes goes undetected.

So what can you do if you get the disease? For starters, keep doing what you've already been doing. Make healthful food choices, stay active, and continue managing your weight. Because you've already developed positive lifestyle habits, you're one step ahead of the game. To fine-tune your routine and to learn more about diabetes, follow up with your health care provider on a regular basis. You'll also want to see a registered dietitian to review your eating habits and follow up with a certified diabetes educator to learn more about diabetes management.

Some organizations that can help you find more information or locate qualified health professionals near you are the American Diabetes Association, the American Association of Diabetes Educators, and the American Dietetic Association. You can also contact local hospitals to find out about support groups for people with diabetes.

It's true that there's always a chance you'll get diabetes even with the perfect plan to prevent it. But don't let this get you down. By making consistent, small changes, you *can* lower your odds of getting diabetes.

SIMPLE CHANGES JOURNAL

What small changes can you make *today* to stay committed to healthy lifestyle behaviors?

What small changes can you make *this week* to stay committed to healthy lifestyle behaviors?

What small changes can you make *this month* to stay committed to healthy lifestyle behaviors?

∿ Bibliography ∿

Part One: Rate Your Risk for Developing Diabetes

Adler, A. I., et al. "The negative association between traditional physical activities and the prevalence of glucose intolerance in Alaska natives." *Diabetic Medicine* 13 (1996): 555–560.

Burke, James P., et al. "Reversion from type 2 diabetes to nondiabetic status: Influence of the 1997 American Diabetes Association Criteria." *Diabetes Care* 21, no. 8 (August 1998): 1266–1270.

"Diabetes facts and figures." American Diabetes Association, 1997. http://www.diabetes.org/ada/c20f.asp [cited 5 Sept. 1999].

"Diabetes risk test." American Diabetes Association, 1999. http://www.diabetes.org/ada/risktest.asp [cited 5 Sept. 1999].

Dornhorst, Anne, and Michela Rossi. "Risk and prevention of type 2 diabetes in women with gestational diabetes." *Diabetes Care* 21, supp. 2 (August 1998): B43–B49.

Helmrich, S. P., et al. "Physical activity and reduced occurrence of non-insulin-dependent diabetes mellitus." *New England Journal of Medicine* 325, no.3 (1991): 147–152.

Manson, J. E., et al. "A prospective study of exercise and incidence of diabetes among US male physicians." *Journal of the American Medical Association* 268, no. 1 (1992): 63–67.

Manson, J. E., and A. Spelsberg. "Primary prevention of non-insulin-dependent diabetes mellitus." *American Journal of Preventive Medicine* 10, no. 3 (1994): 172–184.

Pan, Eizo-Ren, et al. "Effects of diet and exercise in preventing NIDDM in people with impaired fasting glucose tolerance." *Diabetes Care* 20, no. 4 (April 1997): 537–544.

"What you should know about the new report on the diagnosis and classification of diabetes." American Diabetes Association, 1997. http://www.diabetes.ord/ada/newqa.htm [cited 24 June 1997].

Part Two: Make Lifestyle Changes That Last

Labat, Jackie, and Annette Maggi. *Weight Management for Type II Diabetes: An Action Plan.* Minneapolis: Chronimed Publishing, 1997.

Prochaska, James, John Norcross, and Carlo DiClemente. *Changing for Good.* New York: Avon Books, 1994.

Part Three: Manage Your Weight

Bruce, Bonnie, and Denise Wilfley. "Binge eating among the overweight population: A serious and prevalent problem." *Journal of the American Dietetic Association* 96, no. 1 (January 1996): 58–61.

Gibbs, W. Wyat. "Gaining on Fat." *Scientific American,* August 1996: 88–94.

Labat, Jackie, and Annette Maggi. *Weight Management for Type II Diabetes: An Action Plan.* Minneapolis: Chronimed Publishing, 1997.

"Position of the American Dietetic Association: Weight management." *Journal of the American Dietetic Association* 97, no. 1 (January 1997): 71–74.

Part Four: Real Nutrition for Real People

Labat, Jackie, and Annette Maggi. *Weight Management for Type II Diabetes: An Action Plan.* Minneapolis: Chronimed Publishing, 1997.

Tribole, Evelyn, and Elyse Resch. *Intuitive Eating.* New York: St. Martin's Press, 1995.

Part Five: Get Moving, Get Fit

Mayer-Davis, E. J., et al. "Intensity and amount of physical activity in relation to insulin sensitivity—the insulin resistance atherosclerosis study." *Journal of the American Medical Association* 279, no. 9 (1998): 669–674.

Physical Activity and Health: A Report of the Surgeon General. Pittsburgh: U.S. Department of Health and Human Services, U.S. Centers for Disease Control and Prevention, 1996.

"Position Stand of the American College of Sports Medicine: The recommended quantity and quality of exercise for developing and maintaining cardiorespiratory and muscular fitness, and flexibility in healthy adults." *Medicine & Science in Sports & Exercise* 30, no. 6 (1998): 975–991.

Rice, B., et al. "Effects of Aerobic or Resistance Exercise and/or Diet on Glucose Tolerance and Plasma Insulin Levels in Obese Men." *Diabetes Care* 22, no. 5 (May 1999): 684–691.

Part Six: Balance Your Lifestyle

Fanning, Patrick. *Visualization for Change.* Oakland, CA: New Harbinger Publications, Inc., 1994.

Labat, Jackie, and Annette Maggi. *Weight Management for Type II Diabetes: An Action Plan.* Minneapolis: Chronimed Publishing, 1997.

The Life Balance Pyramid. Minneapolis: Park Nicollet HealthSource, 1997.

Teddler, Helen Ashton, and Marlene Johnson. *The Buddy Diet: How Two of You Can Keep It Off Together.* New York: Warner Books, Inc., 1992.

Part Seven: Make Diabetes Prevention a Family Affair

Barth, Joan C. *It Runs in My Family.* New York: Brunner/Mazel, Inc., 1993.

Krause, Carol. *How Healthy Is Your Family Tree?* New York: Simon & Schuster, 1995.

Part Eight: Staying on Track with Your Diabetes Prevention Plan

Baker, Raymond C., and Danieal S. Kirschenbaum. "Self-monitoring may be necessary for successful weight control." *Behavior Therapy* 24 (1993): 377–394.

Prochaska, James, John Norcross, and Carlo DiClemente. *Changing for Good.* New York: Avon Books, 1994.

∿ Index ∾